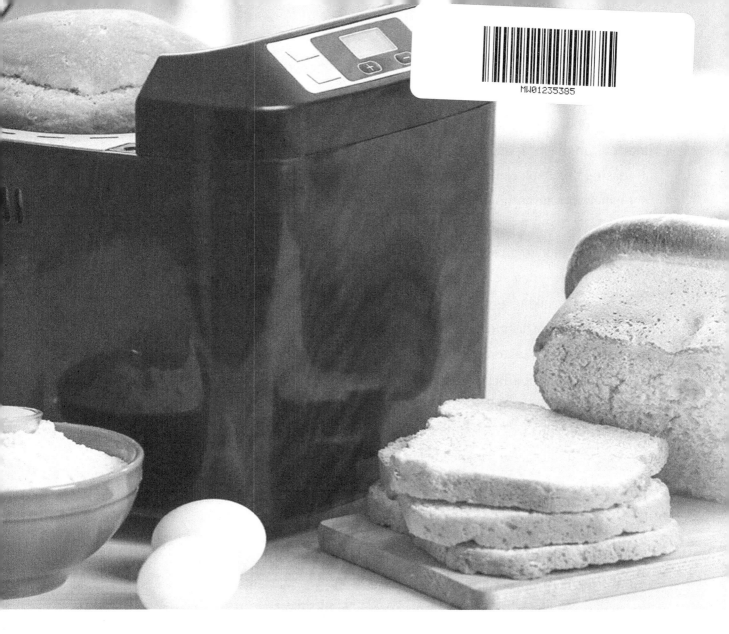

# KETO BREAD MACHINE

THE ULTIMATE STEP-BY-STEP COOKBOOK WITH 101 QUICK AND EASY KETOGENIC BAKING RECIPES FOR COOKING DELICIOUS LOW-CARB AND GLUTEN-FREE HOMEMADE LOAVES IN YOUR BREAD MAKER

*Amanda White*

© Copyright 2020 by Amanda White - All rights reserved.

The Book is reproduced below with the goal of providing information that is as accurate and reliable as possible. Regardless, purchasing this Book can be seen as consent to the fact that both the publisher and the author of this book are in no way experts on the topics discussed within and that any recommendations or suggestions that are made herein are for entertainment purposes only. Professionals should be consulted as needed prior to undertaking any of the actions endorsed herein.

This declaration is deemed fair and valid by both the American Bar Association and the Committee of Publishers Association and is legally binding throughout the United States.

Furthermore, the transmission, duplication or reproduction of any of the following work, including specific information, will be considered an illegal act irrespective of if it is done electronically or in print. This extends to creating a secondary or tertiary copy of the work or a recorded copy and is only allowed with express written consent from the Publisher. All additional right reserved.

The information in the following pages is broadly considered to be a truthful and accurate account of facts, and as such, any inattention, use or misuse of the information in question by the reader will render any resulting actions solely under their purview. There are no scenarios in which the publisher or the original author of this work can be in any fashion deemed liable for any hardship or damages that may occur after undertaking the information described herein. Additionally, the information in the following pages is intended only for informational purposes and should thus be thought of as universal. As befitting its nature, it is presented without assurance regarding its prolonged validity or interim quality. Trademarks that are mentioned are done without written consent and can in no way be considered an endorsement from the trademark holder.

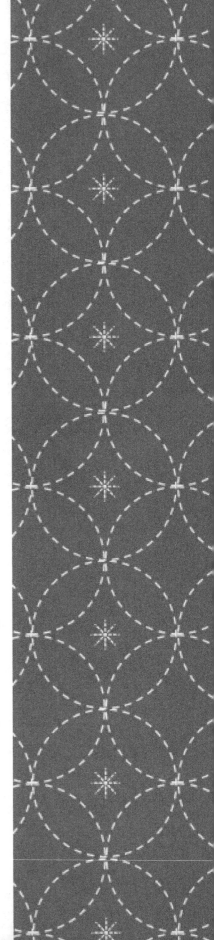

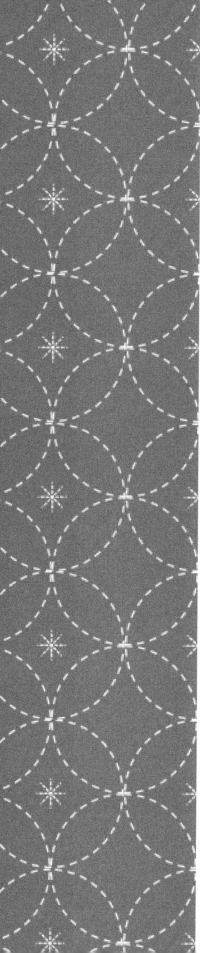

# TABLE OF CONTENTS:

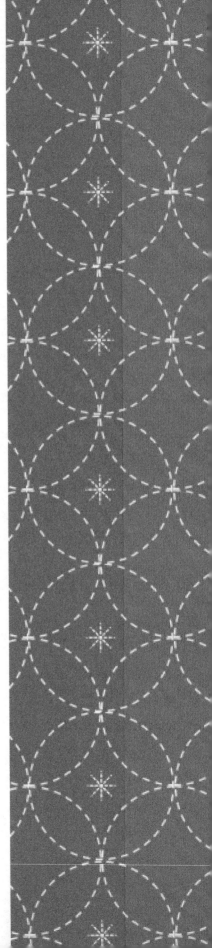

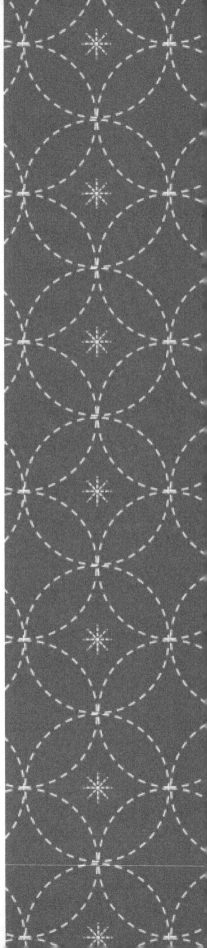

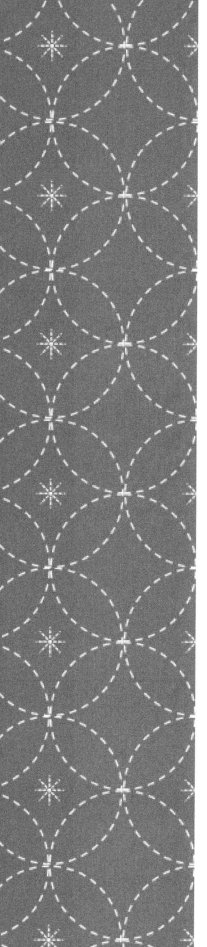

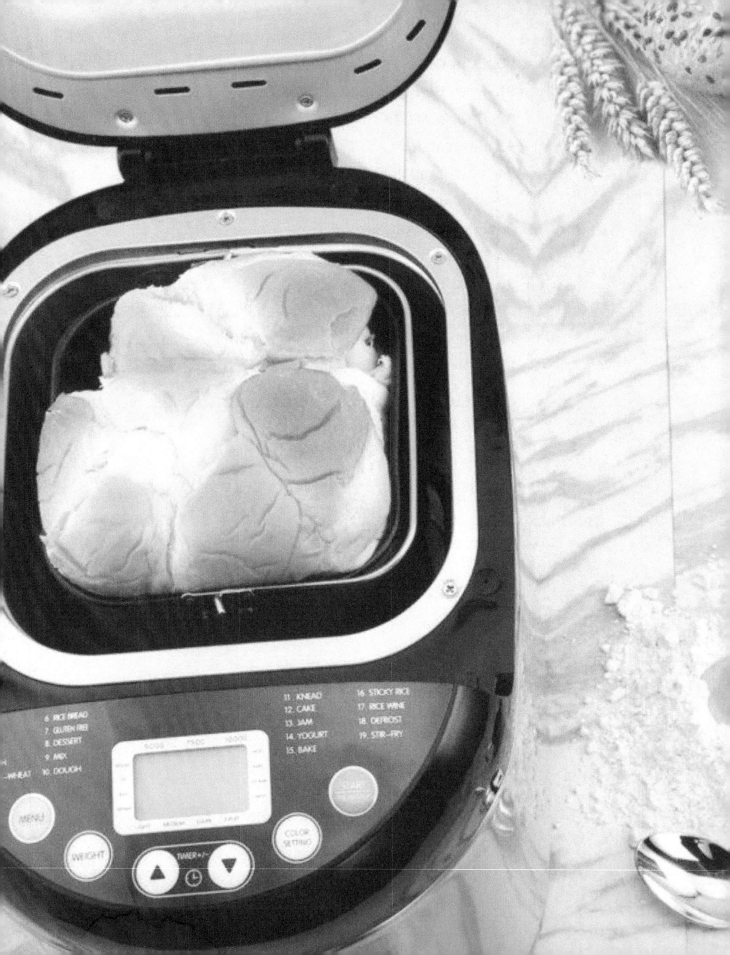

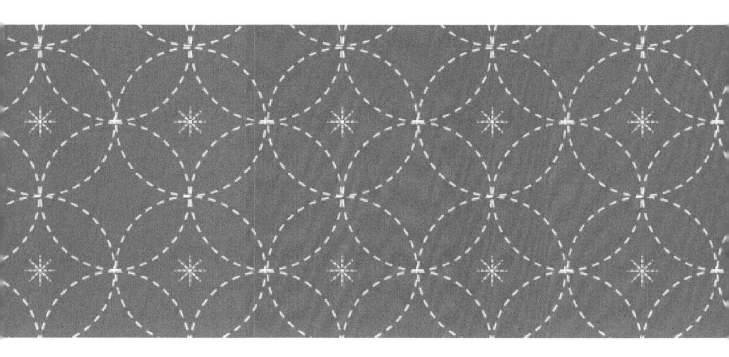

# INTRODUCTION

Bread machine, also known as bread maker, a type of appliance that turns ingredients into baked bread. It comes with a bread pan at the bottom, which looks like paddles in a pizza oven. The bread machine is often controlled by a display panel.

The first bread maker was founded in Japan in 1986 by Panasonic. The purpose of this machine was to train the head bakers to knead bread. As it was industrialized, more companies started creating their own version of the bread machine. Some added a cooling fan at the bottom to allow the machine to cool off after use. Not too long after, it became famous in the United States, Europe, and Australia.

The bread machine is an all-in-one appliance. It takes the guesswork out of making bread by mixing, kneading, proving, and baking the dough. Usually, the bread machine takes a few hours to make a loaf.

Once done, the pan is removed from the bread-maker, which leaves a small hole on the rod where the paddle is attached. Do not be put off by the odd shape of the bread from the machine. It is normal to produce vertical, square, or cylindrical loaves, which is very different from commercialized loaves.

The bread machine is considerably smaller in size than the standard oven. And the usage is defined by the capacity of the bread machine itself. In most cases, the bread machine can accommodate up to 1.5 pounds or 700 grams of dough. There are also bread machines that can accommodate up to 900 grams of dough.

The typical bread maker comes with a built-in timer to control the start and end of the bread-making process. Most machines have a delayed start option, and this allows the bread to start baking even when you are asleep or at work, meaning you'll be greeted by a fresh loaf.

Homemade bread tends to go stale faster than commercial bread as it does not contain any preservatives. There is a natural way to preserve your bread, and it includes using a natural leaven and a pre-ferment in the bread machine. The reason behind this is that it contains a form of lactobacilli. The yeast is responsible for the flavor and the rising of the dough. The lactic acid is responsible for the preservation of the bread.

## Before You Start!

Always remember to check the Directions on your bread machine. It varies across different models and types. So, before you start baking, make sure you know how to program your bread machine for the best quality bread. Your bread machine should come with a timing chart for the different types of bread.

There are bread machines that have their own weighing scale to ensure a proportionate amount of bread inside the machine. Check the capacity of your bread machine.

# Basics About Ketogenic Diet and Bread

After this brief introduction where we have explained what a bread machine is, it is necessary to remember that in this cookbook, we are not going to bake classic bread made with cereal flours but, as you can understand from the title, the recipes will concern the preparation of bread that respects the rules of the ketogenic diet. In the first chapter, I'll explain in detail what the ketogenic diet is, but below I'll give you some quick tips to understand the subject of this cookbook. Probably you already know that the ketogenic diet is one of the most effective forms of weight loss. It helps you burn more fat using a diet that is high-fat and low-carbohydrates. The term "keto" originates from the "ketones" produced by the body when you are in ketosis. When you are in ketosis, your body has nothing to burn for fuel, so in place of the normal carbohydrates you consume, your body begins to burn your own excess body fat. When you keep yourself in ketosis long enough, you become "Fat Adapted", which means your body will automatically burn the excess fat.

Now you're probably wondering, "What is this ketogenic bread?" "How can I make it?"

As a staple food, bread is part of your daily meal plan, even if you are in ketosis. However, flour and sugar, as its main ingredient, make bread one of your number one enemy if you are in a keto diet. This does not mean though that you cannot have bread in your keto diet meal plan. As we'll see in chapter two, you can still eat any kind of bread by substituting flour with keto-friendly alternatives like almond flour and coconut flour.

All bread recipes are prepared with the bread machine and baked in the bread maker or, in some limited cases, in the normal kitchen oven.

But before you begin, you need to consider a few things. The ketogenic diet is not for everyone. If you are taking medications, consult your doctor first before engaging in this diet to avoid any complications.

# Things to Keep in Mind as You Use the Recipes

You are probably going to come across a number of ingredients you haven't heard of before. Rest assured that these can be easily found in most local grocery stores. Some of these ingredients include:

Alternative keto-friendly flours, Psyllium Husk or Psyllium Husk Powder, Xanthan Gum, Inulin and others (see Chapter 2).

## *Sugar substitutes*

As we've seen, sugar is not a food that is included in the keto diet. So, it is necessary to find low carb alternatives to replace the sweet taste of normal sugar. Some examples of substitutes that you can use are erythritol, stevia, sucralose, xylitol, and monk fruit sweetener. You will see this ingredient used in many recipes to give it some sweetness. It is also proven to help lower sugar levels in the body, making it a healthy alternative to traditional processed sugar. See Chapter 1 for best information on low-carb sweeteners.

# Chapter 1: Everything You Need to Know About Ketogenic Diet

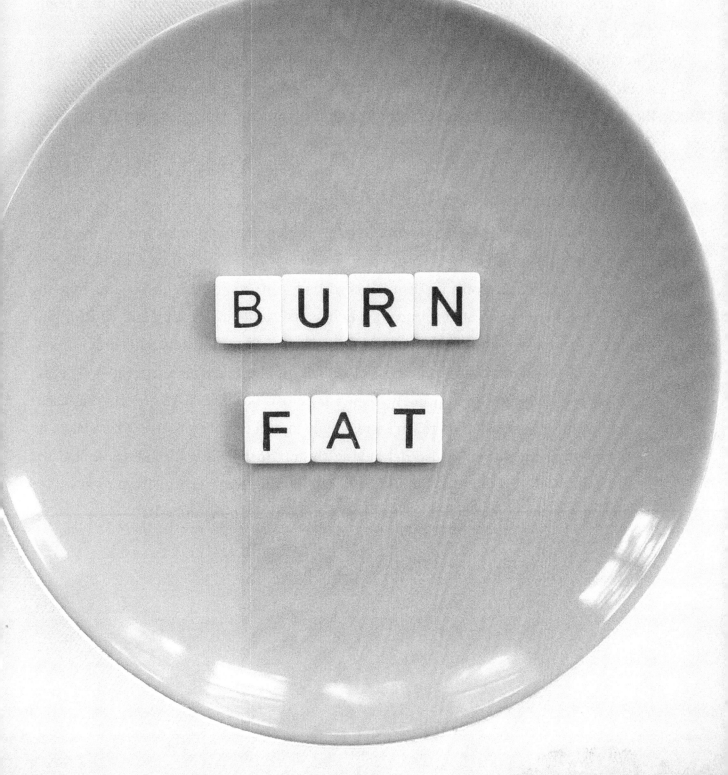

Thanks to the increasing demand for healthy diets and lifestyles, the ketogenic diet has taken center stage. Also known as a low-carb, high-fat meal plan, the keto diet restricts the intake of carbohydrates while promoting healthy fats. Usually, confectioneries and baked goods, snacks, and desserts contain the most carbs since they're predominantly made of sugars and flour. They're also the types of foods that people typically break their diets to eat.

Therefore, this cookbook is full of keto versions of snacks, desserts, and other treats that would normally be forbidden on the low-carb diet. Along with the recipes, you'll also get the ultimate ketogenic guidelines that explain basic information on ketogenic-friendly flours and sweeteners.

## The Ketogenic Diet: Basic Concepts

After years of research and experimentation, scientists and nutritionists worked together to come up with an efficient formula that would not only treat mental illnesses like Alzheimer's and Parkinson's disease but also had a broad impact on general human health. This diet plan created miraculous effects like reducing obesity and controlling insulin in diabetic patients. It eventually came to be known as the ketogenic diet.

The word "keto" comes from the process of ketosis—a physical reaction in the body that this diet produces when appropriately followed. Ketosis is a metabolic process that uses stored fats for energy when there isn't enough glucose in the body to use. This makes it ideal for losing weight while also debunking the myth that fats in food are linked to weight gain. With this diet, the human body can harness more energy from food while producing ketones (a product of ketosis) that detoxify the blood and mind.

In order for any of this to work properly, you have to cut your carb intake using ketogenic carb recommendations. The main carb restriction states that your intake per meal should be no more than 13 grams of carbs. It also requires you to go to embrace high-fat foods instead. Combine this with regular exercise, and you can see the weight loss results you desire. To reduce carbohydrates in your diet, you'll need to remove or limit high-carb ingredients like all grains, lentils, legumes, potatoes, yams, yellow squash, sugars, honey, high-carb fruits, syrups, and the like. You can either avoid them or replace them with low-carb alternatives.

If a person successfully follows the ketogenic diet for about three to four weeks, they can witness marked changes in their physical and mental health. An obese person can lose about two to three pounds in this time period, and a diabetic patient can experience stable insulin levels. People with mental ailments can feel better control over their nerves and emotions, too. Following this diet and lifestyle over a long period of time can even decrease your risk of cancer and complicated cardiac diseases. Cholesterol levels can also be maintained following the ketogenic diet.

## What to Eat and What Not to Eat on a Ketogenic Diet

Eating foods high in fat and low in carbs may sound simple, but it is more difficult to practically implement this idea if you are not familiar with the basics of nutrients. To help you, here is some brief insight regarding all the foods that are restricted and allowed on the ketogenic diet.

First, here are keto-friendly foods to add to your menu:

All dairy and plant fats are ideal for the ketogenic diet. This includes all forms of plants, oils, butter, ghee, cream, and cheese.

All dairy products except milk are suitable for a ketogenic diet. Since milk contains high traces of carbohydrates, it is restricted. When milk is processed to produce yogurt, cream cheese, cream, and other cheeses, the carbs are broken down, making them keto-friendly.

All vegetables low in carbs are allowed on the ketogenic diet, including all greens, above-ground vegetables, onions, garlic, ginger, and similar vegetables.

While most fruits should be limited or avoided, all berries and similar fruits are keto-friendly.

All sugar-free chocolates, sauces, and syrups are safe to use on a ketogenic diet. Ketogenic sugar substitutes are allowed.

Nut-based milk like almond milk, coconut milk, hemp milk, soy milk, etc. are also low-carb and, thus, safe to use.

While knowing what you can eat is great, knowing what not to eat on the ketogenic diet should be your major focus. First, get into the habit of reading labels and nutrition facts for every food you buy to make yourself comfortable with looking for carbs in food. You can't expect to control your carb intake without reading labels. Then, follow this list of high-carb ingredients while grocery shopping and keep them out of your kitchen.

All grains, legumes, lentils, and beans are rich in carbohydrates, so avoid them in any form. Rice, wheat, barley, oats, chickpeas, kidney beans, corn, sorghum, etc. are all a part of this category, too.

Potatoes, yams, beets, yellow squash, and similar vegetables are considered starchy vegetables and are high in carbs and should be avoided.

Apples, bananas, peaches, pears, melons, watermelons, mangoes, pineapples, and similar fruits are all carb-rich and are not allowed on the ketogenic diet.

Any amount of animal milk is restricted. Replace that with nut-based milk.

Flours from grains and lentils like wheat flour, all-purpose flours, and chickpea flour should be avoided and replaced with nut-based gluten-free flours.

White sugars, brown sugars, sugary syrups and beverages, maple syrups, honey, and dates are all forbidden on a ketogenic diet. Replace them with ketogenic sweeteners to add sweetness.

All processed foods with traces of carbohydrates need to be avoided.

# Types of Gluten-Free Ketogenic Flours

Flours are an essential component of all baked desserts, bread, and confectioneries, so they can't be altogether avoided. Since grain- and lentil-based flours are not suitable for the ketogenic diet, look to other gluten-free options to produce the same products with a lower carb content. We will treat in more detail about these alternative flours in Chapter 2.

# Low-carb Sweeteners

Sweeteners play an essential part in building the right balance of flavor in baked desserts. It's not just cakes or cookies that need sweeteners. Almost all desserts from custard to mousses, fat bombs, and ice creams need an excellent sweetener. Since sugar is not an option on a ketogenic diet, you should rely on other low-carb substitutes that are specially manufactured for such a diet. Those substitutes mainly include:

## *Stevia*

Stevia is the strongest of all and tastes 200 times sweeter than ordinary white sugar. It should be used in minimal amounts. It is available in a range of varieties, including powdered and liquid form. Be extra careful while adding this intense sweetener to your recipes or use it as a blend with erythritol. One cup of sugar can be replaced with a teaspoon of stevia powder to get the same sweetness. Stevia is completely natural and comes from the stevia plant, so it doesn't have any adverse effects on your health. It has zero impact on blood sugar and is a great source of magnesium, zinc, potassium, vitamin B3.

## Erythritol

Erythritol, a sugar alcohol produced naturally in fruits and from fermentation, is an exceptional natural and healthy low-carb sweetener that has bulking properties, which make it perfect for baking. Erythritol is a sweetener that leaves no aftertaste, and it is also easy on the stomach. Erythritol and erythritol blends can be used in keto snacks and desserts. Since erythritol has a sweetness level close to that of ordinary sugar, it is more commonly used for ketogenic desserts. As you'll see in the chart below, its conversion is simpler than stevia, too. Another plus point for erythritol is that it contains an extremely low amount of Calories. Where one gram of sugar has around four Calories, the same amount of erythritol contains only 0.24 Calories. Erythritol is available in a powdered form and can be used easily in baking.

## Xylitol

Xylitol is also a naturally occurring sugar alcohol that can be used to sweeten ketogenic desserts. This is probably due to the taste and texture of this natural sweetener. It comes from plants like fruits and vegetables. Xylitol contains anti-bacterial properties that protect the mouth from bacteria that cause tooth decay. Due to its health benefits and curing powers, it is also added to medicines and mints to keep the gums and breath fresh. It is not only low in carbohydrates, but it contains few Calories and ranks very low on the glycemic index.

However, use Xylitol is small quantities to avoid gastrointestinal discomfort. Remind also to keep this product away from dogs because it is toxic to dogs.

## Sorbitol

Another sugar alcohol, sorbitol, is found in several fruits, and it is also present in corn syrup. It is also known as a nutritive sweetener since it can provide as many as 2.6 kcals per gram. Like xylitol, it is also great for sweets, candies, mints, gummies, and bites. It has other medicinal properties that make it good for older people. Whether it's keto or any other diet, the use of this sweetener is always good for your health. It is 60 percent the sweetness of sugar, so 1 cup of sugar can be replaced with 1 ¼ cups of sorbitol.

## Miscellaneous Sweeteners

In recent years, with the diffusion of low carbohydrate diets, a considerable number of sweetening blends have appeared on the market with the aim of replacing classic sugar. Below are some of the best known that we will use in the recipes of this cookbook:

### Swerve

Swerve is a blend of oligosaccharides and erythritol; it is a natural and healthy low carb sweetener that has zero impact on blood sugar. Swerve is another ketogenic sweetener not only used in baking, but also for ice creams, mousses, fat bombs, and other desserts. Swerve is available in all forms, including powder, granulated, white, and even brown, making it perfect for adding texture to different baked items. It can also be added into tea or coffee with no aftertaste and can also be used to cook. Swerve can be used to replace sugar in any recipe, as the same amounts of sugar and swerve have equal sweetness.

### Natvia

Natvia, a blend of stevia and erythritol, is also a natural sweetener. Natvia eliminates the intense aftertaste of stevia, yet retaining its sweetness and combining it with the bulking properties of erythritol to make a perfect healthy low carb sweetener suitable for baking.

### Monk Fruit

Monk fruit sweetener is another good option to sweeten your ketogenic desserts and to give them pleasant taste and texture.

# Conversion Chart

Below is a handy conversion table to make the replacement between white sugar and low carb sweeteners in an easy way:

| SUGAR | 1 TSP | 1 TBSP | 1/4 CUP | 1/3 CUP | 1/2 CUP | 1 CUP |
|---|---|---|---|---|---|---|
| **Erythritol** | 1 1/4 tsp | 1 Tbsp + 1 tsp | 1/3 cup | 1/3 cup + 2 Tbsp | 2/3 cup | 1 1/3 cup |
| **Xylitol** | 1 tsp | 1 Tbsp | 1/4 cup | 1/3 cup | 1/2 cup | 1 cup |
| **Swerve** | 1 tsp | 1 Tbsp | 1/4 cup | 1/3 cup | 1/2 cup | 1 cup |
| **Stevia** | - | - | 3/16 tsp | 1/4 tsp | 3/8 tsp | 3/4 tsp |
| **Liquid Stevia** | 3/8 tsp | 3/8 tsp | 1 1/2 tsp | 2 tsp | 3 tsp | 2 Tbsp |
| **Sukrin** | 1 tsp | 1 Tbsp | 1/4 cup | 1/3 cup | 1/2 cup | 1 cup |

## *Sugar Alcohols Glycemic Index*

They are considered dietary fibers due to their chemical composition.

The glycemic index of a food is used to determine if it's suitable for the ketogenic diet. Since sugar has the highest glycemic value 60, all other sweeteners are compared to this value to calculate their glycemic values. Here is a list of commonly used sugar alcohols along with their glycemic values:

| Sugar Alcohols | Glycemic Index |
|---|---|
| Xylitol | 12 |
| Glycerol | 5 |
| Sorbitol | 4 |
| Lactitol | 3 |
| Isomalt | 2 |
| Mannitol | 2 |
| Erythritol | 1 |

# Benefits of Ketogenic Diet

The Keto diet is famous not only because you are able to lose weight fast but also because it has many other benefits. Changing your eating habits will positively affect your body. Not only will you look good, but your body will feel good, too! You will start noticing changes in your body within the first week or two of being on this diet. Eliminating the toxins, you were used to ingesting will make a difference. The list below is not comprehensive by any means but will give you a good idea of what benefits that the Keto diet has to offer aside from the sought-out weight loss that the Keto diet is known for. Almost everyone will see significant improvements from the diet, whether it be from the list below or from other things that have not been mentioned. Since we are all different, and our bodies all react differently, you may experience things that others may or will not experience.

The following list is what I have thought to be profound benefits that the Keto diet has to offer.

## Nonalcoholic Fatty Liver Disease

Nonalcoholic fatty liver disease is a disease when your liver stores too much in its cells. The fat cells that the liver stores are not related to actual fat but to carbs. The livers transform the carbs into triglycerides and store them as fat. This disease affects people of all ages who are at risk of being overweight or obese, have high blood pressure, have type 2 diabetes, to name a few. This disease could potentially have no sign or symptom, but some people have reported fatigue and pain in their upper right abdomen, spider-like blood vessels, jaundice (the yellowing of the skin) and edema (swelling of the legs). Since the possible warning signs are linked to other ailments, there are often other tests that your doctor may have you take, such as blood and imaging test.

Potential complications from this disease are the liver swelling. This swelling can cause scarring, which could potentially lead to liver or even liver failure. There are no medications to help this condition as of yet, but the Keto diet has helped countless people remove the carbs that their diets once had, therefore, lowering the triglycerides. The fat cells do not build up, but instead, the liver uses it as energy. In some cases, people who have had scarring on their livers show a significant improvement because the body is essentially going through a rejuvenation process that will lead to a healthy you!

## High Blood Sugar

We have sugar in our blood. The correct amounts are vital because sugar causes our body's cells and organs to obtain the energy we need to survive. If your body receives too much sugar, instead of having an abundance of energy, you start to feel unwell. Your body cannot break down as much of the overflow of sugar, and this is why you start feeling the symptoms of high blood sugar. You feel drowsy, tired, have blurred vision, headaches, you have a hard time concentrating, tend to be thirsty, having to urinate quite often, to name a few. These are short-term complications for having high blood sugar. Long-term complications can possibly include a heart attack or stroke, kidney failure and nerve problems. There are many causes of having high blood pressure. Your medical professional is able to diagnose long-term issues with high blood pressure as type 1 or 2 diabetes and, in some cases, gestational diabetes. Diabetes is caused when your body is unable to make insulin, or there is not enough insulin to break down any sugar produced by carbs.

Gestational diabetes only occurs in women who are pregnant. Being on the Keto diet will help you be able to manage your diabetes by eliminating the carbs that are not able to be broken down by the insulin. You may also be able to reduce the medications you are prescribed. The lack of carbs in your system will make it easier for your body's functions.

## Improved Digestion

Many of us have a problem with our digestive systems. From diarrhea, IBS (irritable bowel syndrome), constipation, and heartburn. We have all had at least three of these once in our lives. Constipation usually occurs when you are not eating enough fiber or not drinking enough water, among other things. On the opposite end, there is diarrhea. This can be caused by multiple things as well as consuming artificial sweeteners, or certain additives. Acid reflux or heartburn is caused by stomach fluids backing up into your esophagus. Different types of foods can cause this back up, especially if they are fatty or fried foods.  Being overweight also has a high risk of heartburn. IBS or irritable bowel syndrome affects your large intestine. The symptoms for it are bloating, gas, cramping. Diarrhea or constipation. The triggers of IBS include but aren't limited to certain fatty foods, i.e., deep-fried and carbonated drinks. Removing all the fired, greasy and carbonated drinks from your diet will help you improve your digestion. Everyone can benefit from the Keto diet because we all have experienced digestive problems at one time or another. The Keto diet helps you stay on track to avoid all these foods and stick to the healthy ones that will not cause all the above-stated issues.

## Lowering Triglycerides

Triglycerides, as stated before, are a type of fat found in your body. If you have high triglycerides, you are at risk for your arteries to harden, which dramatically increases your risk of a stroke, heart attack or heart disease. Your medical professional has probably checked your levels at one point with a "lipid panel". This is how they diagnosis this. If you focus on what you eat and exercise, you will have a better chance of lowering them. Avoiding sugar and refined carbs can increase these levels. In addition, eating foods with Trans fats or hydrogenated oils or fats can increase levels as well. Focusing on healthier fats such as red meat and fish will help combat high levels. If you are prescribed medications for high triglycerides, the medication and an improvement in your diet should help reduce those dangerous high levels.

## Depression

Depression is categorized as a mood disorder that causes a constant feeling of sadness. It also causes people to lose interest in things they once loved. This mood disorder is a constant in your life, and you cannot one day wake up and be a happier you. Some symptoms of depression include hopelessness, anger, and frustration, being tired all the time, having no energy, trouble thinking, and anxiety feeling of guilt and sleep disturbances. There are still studies conducted on what exactly causes depression, but so far, research has shown that what can lead to depression may be brain chemistry and how neurotransmitters react with other chemicals that should create mood stability.

Some other studies have shown that it might be an inherited trait. A blood relative might have passed down a gene with this particular trait that lacks the function to balance out your moods. Your body needs to be able to convert glutamate (a transmitter that your body has to get "messages" to the brain; you're welcome! I didn't know what this was either!) Into GABA (this is the body's main neurotransmitter). You need the right balance of both to have your brain function normally. When you are on a high carb diet, your brain isn't able to convert enough glutamate to GABA. This means that your body is suffering from neurotoxicity. Having your body goes into Ketosis, it seems to encourage the balance of both glutamate and GABA, which alleviates the symptoms of depression.

## Acne

Acne, as many of us know, is a skin condition that starts from adolescence during puberty and sometimes follows us into our adult life. The root cause of acne is when a pore in your skin becomes clogged, bacteria, excess of the androgens hormone, or excess oil production. There are different types of acne, which include whiteheads, blackheads, and pimples (zits). They can appear on your face, forehead, chest upper back, and shoulders. We know how slightly they can be and sometimes painful! There are many myths surrounded by what affects acne, such as the makeup you wear, hygiene and eating greasy foods. One of the actual triggers that can lead to acne is your diet.

Eating too many carbohydrate-rich foods. Eating all these carbs can alter your stomach bacteria because you are adding excess sugar to your bloodstream, which can cause inflammation of the skin, among other things. If you reduce your intake of these carbs, you reduce the risk of inflamed skin. You can also consume more fatty fish that are rich in omega-3, eat the lowest carb-filled vegetables and limit your dairy intake to maximize the benefit.

## Heart Health

Keto can also benefit your heart health! Losing weight and can help you lessen the risk of heart disease. This is two for the price of one! Cardiovascular disease is actually an umbrella term that incorporates various issues that affect your health regarding blood vessels or heart problems. This disease is when your heart is damaged by the buildup of plaque in the heart's major blood vessels. The buildup limits the blood flow to the heart, and this will limit the flow of oxygen as well. Your doctor will typically run a lab test in order to diagnosis you. This disease is very common and affects approximately 3 million people across the United States. CAD can end up weakening the heart muscles, which in turn can cause heart failure. Heart failure is when your heart cannot pump the blood the rest of your body needs. CAD can also cause heart arrhythmias. Heart arrhythmias are changes in the way your heartbeats. Instead of having a steady beat, it is either beating too fast, too slow or irregularly. By reducing the intake of carbs, you can try and reduce or not add any more of the buildup of the fatty deposits that are associated with the CAD.

## Brain Health

Epilepsy is a central nervous system disorder that causes brain activity to become abnormal. There are different types of symptoms, including twitching in the arms or possibly legs, as well as staring out into nothingness for a short period of time with a blank stare. Once you have a seizure, your seizures typically tend to stay the same, and nothing will change drastically. There are many causes of this disorder. A few are head trauma, brain conditions such as tumors or strokes, and injuries to the brain before birth, such as lack of oxygen and developmental disorders.

Your medical will evaluate your symptoms and order a neurological exam, which includes testing motor skills and mental focus as well as blood exams, EEGs, CT scans, MRI, PETs, to name a few. Several studies have shown that the Keto diet has been linked to patients who have seen a reduction in the number of seizure episodes they have. Having the body go into the ketosis stage helps in altering your brain's metabolism to reduce the risk of having seizures. Many experts use the Keto diet as an aid to reduce seizures. Patients are still medicated but are still on the Keto diet to bring out the best outcome for the patient. Studies are being conducted for more brain conditions in hopes of either finding a cure or helping patients live a better life.

## *Migraines*

Migraines are caused when nerve cells are overactive ad send out the incorrect signals to the nerves that are connected to your head and face. Sending these signals causes the chemical to be released and cause the blood vessels in the lining of your brain to swell. This is what causes the unbearable pain you experience when you have a migraine. There are a few triggers for migraines like changes in the weather, changes in your sleeping habits, skipping meals, caffeine, stress, and food. When you suffer from migraines, you typically experience different "stages" before the actual onset of the migraine. Stage 1 is the prodromal stage. The second stage is called the Aura stage. Stage 3 is the Attack stage. The last stage is called the postdrome stage. In the first stage, you experience either high energy or being extremely depressed.

You can also experience cravings, the need to urinate quite often and sleepiness. In the second stage, you start noticing changes in your vision, and you may feel like you are on "pins and needles" and also may have difficulties with speaking or writing. In the third stage, the actual migraine begins. In this stage, you may have a migraine for, hopefully, just a few hours, or it can last for several days. You are sensitive to light, you feel throbbing, and it may only affect one side of your face or, in some cases, your whole face. Some people even have said they experience nausea and vomiting. In the last stage and when the migraine is over, you feel exhausted and sometimes confused.

A study done around 2009 showed that people who were on the Keto diet showed reduced signs of migraines. The researchers were first trying to have the patients lose weight to see if that would help them overall. The patients who were doing the Keto diet were the patients that had experienced the greatest reduction of migraines. They also had their non-overweight patients that suffer from migraines get on the Keto diet as well, and they too had reduced amounts of migraines. Because of the low carbs in the Keto diet, researchers have found that it reduces the migraine, causing inflammation of the blood vessels in the lining of your brain.

## Muscle Mass and Performance

While you are on the Keto diet, you can increase your muscle mass as well. Carbs are not necessary to build the lean muscles some people are looking to create. In order to build muscle, you need to eat enough proteins, eating the calories in healthy fats and you need to weight train. You might gain muscle mass quicker if you are eating carbs, but you need to remember that in eating carbs, you will be eating the unhealthy fats that make you gain weight. If you are looking to maintain the lean muscles that you worked hard for, it is easier to maintain them on the Keto diet because you are losing fat and not your muscle mass. Studies have also shown that the Keto diet doesn't decrease your performance. Your body is just using a different way to energize itself. When you start the Keto diet, you will see a little slowdown in your performance, but this is expected because your body is going through a change that will take time to get adapted to. Once your body has now become accustomed to the way it is now converting fats into ketones, it will go back to where it once was performance-wise. You need to remember, though, to make sure that you are eating enough protein, calories, and training correctly, which are vital. The Keto diet will hurt your body's performance, nor will it hinder you from gaining or maintaining muscle mass. The benefits listed here are just the tip of the iceberg when it comes to all the health benefits that the Keto diet has to offer. Usually, enhanced weight loss is what people think of when they hear "Keto diet." Most are not aware of the vast benefits that are associated with the diet.

A quick non-in depth assessment of other benefits include helping to manage your appetite. It is a way to maintain your weight because your body is always burning your fat; it can help aid in the treatment of metabolic syndrome. It also aids in fighting different diseases, which can include Parkinson's, TBI (Traumatic Brain Injury), and Alzheimer's, to name just a few. Researchers are also starting to look into how the Keto diet may help with the possible removal of sugar consumption and replace it in hopes of killing off the cancer cells.

You will also feel more energized. Who doesn't want to feel this way!? Since your cutting the dreaded carbs, you will not be getting the effects of the sugar rushes that your body was used to, and you will always have that steady source of energy and not the sporadic one that we all wish would last for days. You will see a significant change in your overall mood and memory. Since you are eliminating ingredients that are not natural, your body will only be processing foods that it should be, therefore not sending out unhealthy toxins that affect your mood and memory. Wouldn't it be nice to remember where you placed your keys instead of looking for them for about ten minutes before you realize they are in your hands? No? Was that just me?

The Keto diet will also help with recovering faster from exercise. Deciding to add that extra five or ten pounds to your training regimen and dreading the next few days because of the achy and sore muscles will be a thing of the past. You will be able to recover faster because your body will not be as inflamed because of the reduction of carbs.

# CHAPTER 2:   MAIN INGREDIENTS TO USE TO PREPARE KETOGENIC BREAD

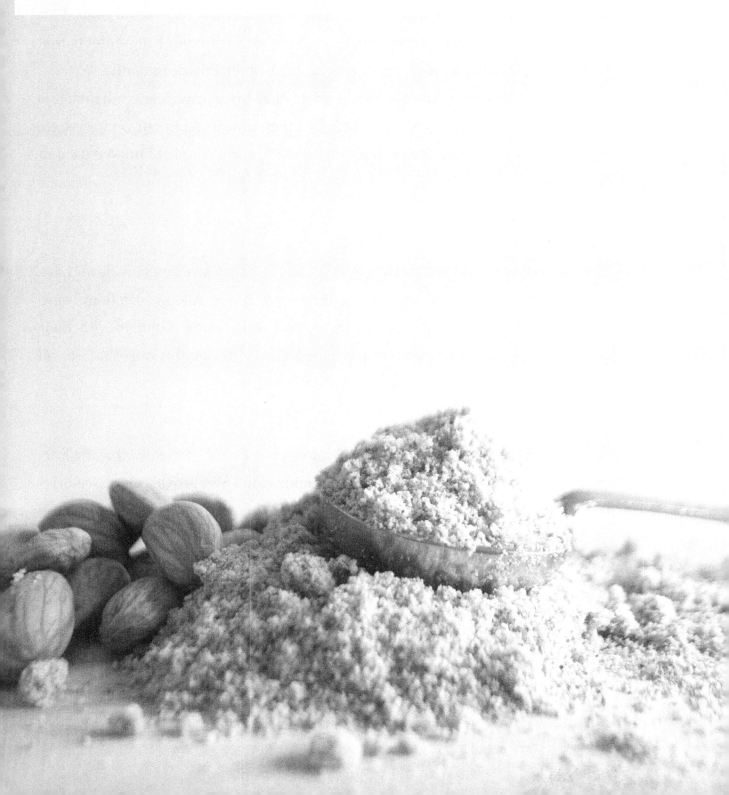

Enjoying the best flavors and textures of our baked bread ought to be more than having something to fold around a burger, satisfy your hungry appetite, or satisfying your cravings with excessive empty calories. I'm sure you must have heard about completely abstaining from bread if you want to live the Keto lifestyle, well I am happy to let you know that keto bread can now be an exciting addition to your daily nutritional goals. This is because, unlike your regular bread, keto bread is made with unique ingredients that uphold the law of keto dieting, which is low carbs, high-fat diet predominantly.

Even though we shall be spending our hard-earned cash on expensive ingredients, it is essential to know where they originate from, what they contribute to our body system, and how they help us. Here are the primary ingredients, and a couple of minors used in Keto bread making.

## Ketogenic Flour Alternatives

Using low carb flours can be overwhelming for you at first because you may never have used them. Low carb flours don't really work like regular flours. All low carb flours have their peculiarity, and as you get used to them, you will become familiar with their characteristics and how best to use them in recipes. The keto-friendly flours that we will use most for the recipes in this cookbook are the following:

### *Almond flour*

This flour comes from almonds finely ground into a powder and is used for baking low-carb bread and desserts. It is rich in minerals, vitamins, and also provides more calories than other nuts. Almond flours are made by blanching almonds to remove the skins and then grinding them until a fine floury-consistency is reached. ¼ cup or about 28g almond flour contains 160 Calories and 3g net carbs. Store almond flour in a well-lidded container and keep refrigerated after opening. The rules you need to follow are given below:

- Use only dried or fresh almonds.
- Grind a small number of almonds at a time.

- Don't grind a portion for over thirty seconds.
- Slightly shake the blender or grinder as you go.

Most almond flour brands are more coarsely ground, which influences the final texture in baked products. In thick or brisk-type bread, this doesn't generally make a difference. However, when we're trying to achieve more tender loaf— white bread, Challah, French-style—the appearance and taste response are important. Search for brands that show they are finely ground.

They are pricier, but you will be more joyful with the finished product.

## *Almond Meal*

Almond meal, also known as ground almonds, has the same amount of macros as the almond flour and contains the same amounts of minerals and vitamins. The difference between almond meal and almond flour is the absence of blanching. The almonds are ground with their skin-on until a slightly rough consistency is reached. It can be used in many baking recipes as an alternative to almond flour. Almond meal can be likened to the consistency of cornmeal. But almond meal is not the same as almond flour. Meal is coarser and not ideal for every bread, dessert, or confectionery. Instead, it's only used when you need a crumbly texture for a recipe. Keep this differentiation in your mind when choosing ingredients; don't substitute one for the other.

The almond meal should also be stored in a well-lidded container and refrigerated after opening.

## Coconut Flour

Coconut flour is another low-carb flour that is very high in fiber and protein and, as the name indicates, comes from the dehydrated white flesh of a coconut. It is so finely ground that it turns into flour and gives a nice texture and taste to recipes. The texture of coconut flour is not exactly like wheat flour; it is denser and can soak up more moisture than wheat flour. Due to this, extra water or liquid needs to be added to give coconut flour the same texture batters or doughs. The ability to absorb more moisture is one of the characteristics of coconut flour. This flour can also make lots of clumps in a batter; use a good beater or whisk your mixtures well with a fork to break up any clumps.

As a beginner, do not do without the extra moisture, butter, or eggs you find in recipes. 2 tbsp or 18 g coconut flour contains 45 Calories and 2 net carbs.

Store coconut flour in a well-lidded container or sealed bag and keep it in a dark pantry out of direct sunlight.

Advantages of coconut flour are given below:

- Coconut flour is rich in protein, fiber, and iron.
- The protein content in the coconut flour is comparable or higher than in whole-grain wheat.
- The coconut flour does not have the distinctive exotic taste like coconut butter, cream, and milk.

Disadvantages of coconut flour:

- The high-fiber content can cause a problem for some types of bread.

Secrets of cooking with coconut flour:

- Always sift the flour before using it.
- Mix dough more thoroughly than with usual flour.
- Watch the baking time.

## White Bean Flour

It has a gentle, smooth nutty flavor and braces our shortlist of useable flours in keto bread making. It contains a one of a kind fiber called resistant starch, which implies that unlike refined carbohydrates that basically melts and blends into our circulatory systems, it goes through the small intestine, for the most part, as undigested fiber. It enhances digestive health by promoting the development of useful microorganisms and manages blood glucose levels because the energy is discharged later in the large intestine, averting sharp spikes and diminishes between meals. Other significant by-products of this flour's digestive process are chemical compounds called "short-chain unsaturated fatty acids," which help counteract colon disease by preventing the absorption of cancer-causing agents (carcinogens). When compared with other flours, it contains the most starches. However, its advantages are more.

## Ground Flaxseed

Flaxseeds are a rich source of healthy fats, vitamins, minerals, and antioxidants, making them quite beneficial for digestion and heart health. Flaxseed flour and meal can both be used in the ketogenic diet.

Flaxseed bread, muffins, and cookie recipes are in this book to give you a simple idea on how to use this super nourishing seed flour or meal. Processed flaxseed flour is available at most grocery stores.

### Flax Meal

Flaxseed or ground flax is very nourishing and a great source of Vitamin B1, Copper, and Omega − 3. Like an almond meal, flaxseed meal is coarser than the ground flaxseed so take that into account when following recipes. Ground flaxseeds are a good alternative for eggs in some baking recipes. Substitute a mixture of 3 tbsp. of water and 1 tbsp. ground flax meal for 1 egg and let sit until moisture is absorbed. This alternative only works for recipes that are not heavily egg-based. 2 tbsp. or 14 g of ground flax meal contains 70 Calories and 1 g Net Carb. To prevent staleness, store flax meal in a well-lidded mason jar and refrigerate or freeze before and after you open it.

### Pumpkin seed/Sunflower seed meal

These flours can conveniently replace almond meal or almond flour in any recipe. You can use a food processor or coffee grinder to make your own homemade pumpkin seed or sunflower meals. Pumpkin and sunflower seeds meal can be stored in a cool, dark pantry for up to 4 months.

# How to replace gluten?

No gluten-free flour, or any blend thereof, can copy the flexibility, gas–holding and binding characteristics of gluten. It does superb, magical things, allowing ease of kneading and stretching, creating superbly chewy, fluffy, and airy bread. Unfortunately, all the ketogenic flours we have seen are gluten-free. This can be appreciated by those who have a gluten intolerance, but its absence is felt when baking baked goods. So what are our other options to replace it?

Egg whites have been a major help; however, something more is needed to achieve the desired texture and suppleness we're searching for.

We have three essential gluten—substitution choices: xanthan gum, psyllium and oat fibers; there's also ground seeds like chia and flaxseeds that become gelatinous when water is added.

## Xanthan Gum

Before we move onto the fun part of baking, you must learn that xanthan gum is going to be your new best friend. You may not realize this, but many of the gluten-free flour alternatives lack a binding agent. A binding agent is helpful to hold your food together, much like gluten does when used in baking and cooking. The moment you remove gluten, all mixtures will typically crumble and fall apart. Xanthan gum is made from lactose, sucrose, and glucose that have been fermented from a specific bacterium. When this is added to liquid, it creates a gum and is used with gluten-free baking. As a general guide, you will be using one teaspoon of xanthan gum for one cup of gluten-free flour that you use. For some mixes, this gum is already added, so when you are baking, you will always want to check the ingredient label. It should be noted that xanthan gum can be expensive, but it will last you a long time.

If you have an allergy to xanthan gum, you can find ways around it. Instead, you can try using psyllium husks, ground flaxseeds, or ground chia seeds. Psyllium can be sold in full husks or powder. As you bake more, you will soon find what works for you and what doesn't!

## Psyllium Husk Powder

This commonly known husk is obtained from the seeds of Plantago ovata. Basically, it is an excellent soluble fiber supplement. Available in both powder and husk form, this supplement is also good for the ketogenic diet. Unflavored psyllium husks are sold both whole and as a ground powder. Powdered psyllium makes for dense bread. Psyllium seed husk helps to produce a bread-like texture, as it replaces gluten to a certain extent. The husk is highly absorbent, so although the bread will not have the same airy texture as gluten-rich bread, its inclusion produces a moisture loaf. There is no carbohydrate content since the husk is pure fiber.

The powder is suitable to use in several ketogenic breads, desserts, and confectioneries as it has a light and airy touch that gives food a fluffy and soft texture.

### Oat fiber

Oat fiber is a powdered fiber. It is pure fiber, not a flour; it is obtained by grinding the skin and shell of oatmeal grains. It should not be confused with oatmeal, which is derived from the grain itself (separated from the peel) and, due to its high carbs content, is not suitable for preparing ketogenic foods.

Practically oat fibers consist only of ground husks and are generally not used as the main ingredient for baking. The product obtained by grinding the hull is made up of over 90% insoluble fibers and is practically free of carbohydrates and calories.

This type of fiber is known to absorb water easily (up to 7 times its weight). This allows it to bind easily to fat and retain moisture, making bakery products more workable. They are, therefore, ideal in addition to the other alternative flours mentioned in this chapter to improve the consistency of the dough.

Oat fibers also help intestinal regularity and are gluten-free.

## Protein Source Ingredients

### Natural Whey Protein Powder

This obviously cannot be described as flour for any reason; however, to make keto bread, it is an incredible substitution. Whey is the fluid that is left after the main phases of cheese production and then processed into a concentrated powder. It is viewed as total protein and contains every one of the nine essential amino acids. Studies have proven that, in addition to improving muscle quality (which helps the muscle to burn more calories), these essential amino acids help avert cardiovascular diseases, diabetes, and age-related bone loss. And there's more—from anti-cancer properties to improving food reaction in kids with asthma. Even though It must be enhanced with our other flours, it breaks down rapidly to help make delectable, healthy, nutrient-rich baked products.

You can find 100% natural unflavored whey protein from health food portions at online stores, and they are likely to be more affordable than the various brands sold in the grocery stores. It is important to search for products without any additives and also consider the brands and costs while shopping.

## Egg Whites

Having lots of egg whites in a recipe are genuinely economical and simple to plan. I get them in two different ways; in powder form in a 36-ounce canister that equals 255 egg whites and; in the fluid form, which can be bought with discounts at stores like Costco or 1-quart containers in nearby staple goods. I have seen wide varieties in cost, so be sure to compare before buying. Since they are pasteurized, they won't whip so well as new whites, however adding a small quantity of cream of tartar will make excellent, fluffy steeps similarly as high as using fresh egg whites.

Egg whites are essentially 90% water and 10% proteins, which are long chains of amino acids. When we beat air into the whites, these chains become denatured, which implies they unwind and stretch into shapes that trap air, making light textures in what we bake. There is a school of thought that heating/cooking protein—which includes protein powders like whey—decimates the nutritional worth because our bodies can't assimilate "denatured" foods. This is false. If that were the case, we would need to eat everything raw, right?! Eggs, meat, all that we cook and prepare are denatured when warmed. The food leaves the stove changed in appearance, yet the protein isn't denatured; rather than being folded into tight molecular balls, the protein chains become long strands.

Cooked or raw, our bodies retain the same essential amino acids. Understanding what denaturing truly is, enables us to appreciate many healthy foods, unhindered by senseless arguments.

# Ingredients for Leavening and Baking

## Yeast

I buy ACTIVE dry yeast in economical 2-pound bundles and store it in a zip–lock bag in the freezer. It just takes two or three minutes for one tablespoon of yeast powder to warm to room temperature. I measure it straight from the freezer, (speedily returning it), regularly adding it to the bowl of dry ingredients without proofing (allowing it to break down and activate it into a froth before adding to the batter).

Yeast production today is very reliable. Proofing is only useful if it is past the expiry date, and you have to test whether it is still good and can be useful. It will activate when it interacts with the fluid fixings in the blending procedure. There is just one rise with low–carb bread. This is my hypothesis, though, however, since yeast has so little to eat—essentially only a tablespoon of Honey—I don't need it to generate the entirety of its energy in a different dish; I need its work to begin inside the batter. I tried this, one loaf with sealed yeast included and the other with the yeast entering the batter dry; the subsequent loaf rose higher. All brand name names of yeast sold in North America are without gluten except for brewer's yeast utilized in lager production.

## Honey

Don't be scared to hear about honey or sugar in a ketogenic cookbook; I'm not crazy. Honey is important to give food to the yeast and activate it since the flours used in keto diet don't contain sugars to eat or starches to convert into glucose. For the same reason, you can use ordinary sugar, if you like. Obviously, just one tablespoon is used for the whole formula and separated into 8, 12, or 16 servings, and our portion is quite small. It should also be remembered that practically all this tablespoon will be used as food by the yeast and will be converted into alcohol and carbon dioxide. So there will be any sugar left in your ketogenic bread. According to the American Diabetes Association, consuming white sugar increases blood glucose levels somewhat quicker than Honey, which has a glycemic run somewhere in the range of 31 and 78 relying upon the variety.

Locust honey, for example, has a glycemic index (GI) of 32; clover honey has 69. You can investigate this further on online sites like the Glycemic Index Database. Local raw nectar additionally seems to help regular sensitivities since the honey bees gather region dust, which helps construct your invulnerability.

If you absolutely do not want to use that spoonful of sugar or honey, you can replace it with Inulin (see below).

## Inulin

This ingredient you will find in most recipes that include yeast. In traditional bread recipes that use yeast, you need to have sugar to feed the yeast, which is what helps your bread double in size. Inulin is a naturally occurring substance that feeds yeast the same way sugar does in recipes.

## Diastatic Malt Powder

Diastatic Malt Powder has, for some time, been a hidden secret of professional bakers. Albeit just one teaspoon is added to every one of the following recipes, it critically enhances the flavor and produces an appetizing home-baked bread aroma. It is listed as a discretionary element for gluten-free diets since it is produced from sprouted grains (for example, barley) that have been dried and ground. Luckily gluten-free varieties of malt and malt substitutes are additionally being created and are accessible on a limited basis. "Diastatic" alludes to the enzymes that are present as the grain newly sprouts, which convert starches into sugars and advances yeast growth.

I have not been able to decide whether these enzymes separate the resistant starches found in white bean flour; I just know the taste and texture are obviously better, and the bread remains fresh for a more extended period. It usually comes in a 1-pound pack that is generally cheap because only one teaspoon is utilized per portion. Note: Do not mistake this for non–diastatic, which is basically a sugar without any enzymes.

# Oils and Fats

Oils rich in saturated fats, for example, corn oil and vegetable oil, are not allowed. Instead, select oils that are high in omega-3s, for example, olive, coconut, and avocado oil.

# Oil And Butter Alternatives

### Coconut Oil

There is a wide range of health benefits obtained from coconut oil. It's beneficial for your heart, your assimilation, and your resistant framework, and is additionally valuable in assisting with weight reduction. It has a light, however particular coconut flavor.

### Almond Butter

Almonds top the chart of the "world's most beneficial foods" list on the earth. Almond butter gives a pleasant nutty flavor, which can be likened to peanut spread in your dishes.

### Cashew Butter

Rich in a few distinct nutrients, cashew butter is additionally high in protein and is a great substitute for butter or nutty spread in a recipe. It does, obviously, have an aftertaste like cashews.

### Macadamia Butter

Macadamia nuts are a rich source of dietary fiber and monounsaturated fats. The butter is sweet and velvety and lessens bad cholesterol in the body while increasing good cholesterol. Macadamia butter is a good substitution for the regular butter and has a sweet, nutty flavor.

# Milk Alternatives

### Almond Milk

Pressed from almond seeds, almond milk is high in protein and low in bad fats. It's a perfect, tasty swap for dairy and has a scarcely recognizable and very mellow flavor.

### Coconut Milk

Pressed from the meat of the coconut, coconut milk keeps up stable glucose and advances cardiovascular, bone, muscle, and nerve wellbeing. It gives a rich, sweet coconut flavor to your dishes.

# Other Ingredients

### Meats and Proteins

Your meats need to come from grass-fed, organically produced livestock, free-range poultry, or wild-caught fish and assorted types of seafood. Wild game is excellent, as well, in case you're so interested. Meats, for example, venison, are very low in bad fats while high in good fats and lean protein, so don't hesitate to get some for yourself!

### Fruits and Vegetables

If it is remotely possible, shop at your nearby ranchers' market for fresh organic fruits and veggies. Since the Paleo diet is dependent upon your inventiveness to finish a hot, new, delicious supper without the aid of flours, fats, and other no-no's, you will need to gain proficiency with various approaches to get ready healthy dishes within the shorts time. In addition, if you're offering a wide assortment of foods that your family knows and cherishes, you won't be under such a great amount of pressure to cook a simple dish that everyone will eat and really appreciate. Tomatoes are great for any serving of mixed greens and make a tasty base for soups and sauces. They're loaded with nutrients and have a great number of uses that you ought to have some close by consistently. Different meals ought to incorporate carrots, peppers, cauliflower, and celery.

For fruits, choose ones that are high in vitamins and generally low in sugar, for example, stone fruits and berries. Berries are likewise great sources of antioxidants, phytonutrients, and minerals. Apples are healthy organic snacks, as are peaches, oranges, and bananas. The dark tip of the banana that you take out is highly rich in Vitamin K, so do your body a huge favor and eat it!

## Seasonings

Your success with making the change to the caveman diet (Paper diet) is, to a great extent, reliant on how delightful your food is. Thus, you're going to need to fuse different herbs and flavors to make your dishes heavenly. Here are a few that you ought to consistently have close by:

- All spice
- Dark pepper
- Basil
- Cayenne pepper
- Cinnamon
- Cloves
- Squashed red pepper
- Curry powder
- Dry mustard
- Garlic (fresh and powdered)
- Mustard seed
- Oregano
- Paprika
- Parsley
- Rosemary
- Thyme

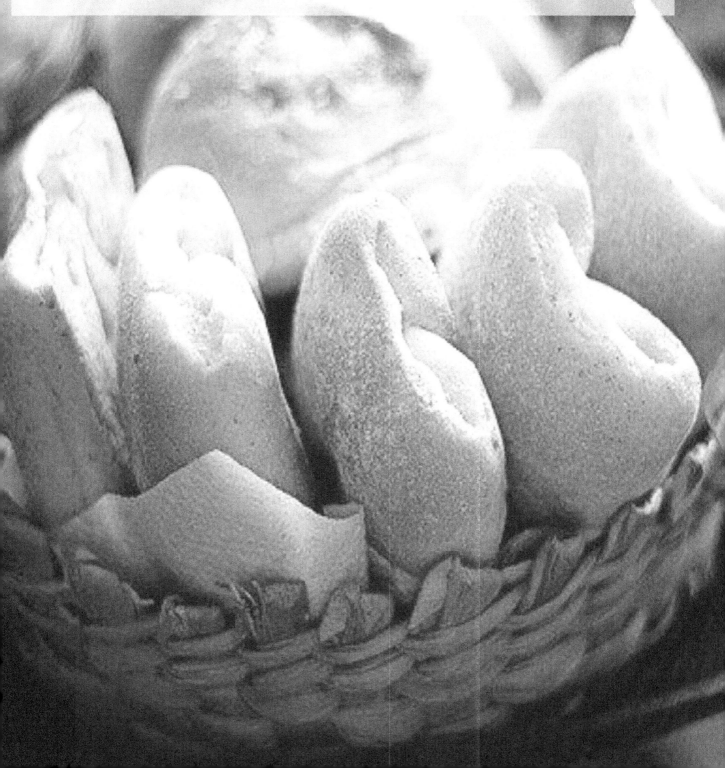

# CHAPTER 3: BRIEF GENERAL EXPLANATION OF MAIN TYPES OF KETO BREAD

A staple food is a food regularly eaten in quantities that make it a predominantly standard diet for some people. Some common staple foods include meat, eggs, fish, cheese, root vegetables or tubers like potatoes and cassava, starchy tubers, and cereals from which bread is made.

## Different Types of Bread

There are many types of bread, but only three categories to which they can be classified. The first is bread that rises high and has to be baked in pans like bread loaves and muffins; the second are breads with medium volume like baguettes, rye bread, and other French bread; and the last are those that hardly rise or more known as flatbread like naan bread, tortilla bread, pizza bread, and crackers.

Some of the most popular breads that people normally eat for breakfast, lunch or dinner include:

### *Loaves*

These are rounded or oblong mass of dough baked in rectangular pans. Loaves come in white bread, multi-grain, brown bread, Ezekiel bread and many others. The loaves are the most common type of bread.

### *Bagels*

Bagel is a type of bread resembling a doughnut, but unlike regular bread, bagels are prepared by boiling first in water before baking.

### *Pizza*

Pizza is a round flatbread topped by tomato sauce, cheese and some added meat and vegetables. The pizza is of Italian origin. Pizza can also be prepared using a loaf bread. Muffins. Muffins are prepared and baked like cakes, but muffins are a type of bread and not cake. Muffins are usually eaten for breakfast and can be sweet or savory.

## Breadsticks

Breadstick is a dry bread that resembles thin-sized pencils in form and normally used as a dipping stick. Breadstick originated from Turin, Italy, and is usually served as an appetizer.

## Crackers

Cracker is a type of bread made from wheat flour and water and comes in many forms like rye and multi-grain.

# CHAPTER 4: WHAT IS A BREAD MACHINE?

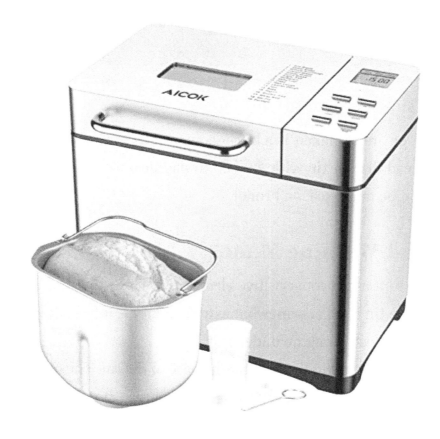

Bread is a baked food that can be set up from various kinds of batter. The mixture is ordinarily made of flour and water. Bread is prepared in several shapes, sizes, types, and surfaces. Extents and kinds of flour and different fixings shift, as do techniques for arrangement. Since the commencement, bread has been one of the most fundamental nourishments, as it is likewise one of the most established counterfeit nourishments. Truth be told, individuals were making bread since the beginning of horticulture.

Individuals in all societies serve bread in different structures with any dinner of the day. It tends to be eaten as a piece of the supper or as a different bite.

## How Do You Cook Bread?

Bread is typically arranged from wheat flour mixture, which is made with yeast and permitted to rise. Normally, individuals heat bread in the stove. In any case, an ever-increasing number of individuals go to the extraordinary bread machines to prepare crispbread at home.

## What Is A Bread Machine?

A bread machine, or bread maker, is a kitchen apparatus for heating bread. The gadget comprises of a bread dish or tin with worked in paddles, which is situated in the focal point of a little unique multi-reason broiler.

## How Is Bread Machine Made?

This machine is essentially a conservative electric appliance that holds a solitary, huge bread tin inside. The tin itself is somewhat extraordinary – it has a hub at the base that is associated with an electric engine underneath.

A little metal oar is appended to the pivot at the base of the tin. The oar is answerable for manipulating the mixture. A waterproof seal secures the hub itself. We should investigate every one of the bread machine parts in detail:

- The top over the bread producer comes either with the survey window or without it
- The control board is likewise situated on the highest point of the bread machine with the end goal of comfort
- In the focal point of the top, there is a steam vent that depletes the steam during the heating procedure. A portion of the bread creators likewise have an air vent on the gadget for air to come inside the tin for the mixture to rise

# How Does Bread Machine Work?

To begin with, you put the plying paddle inside the tin. At the point when the tin is out of the machine, you can gauge the fixings and burden them into the tin.

A while later, you simply need to put the skillet inside the stove (machine), pick the program you wish by means of the electronic board, and close the top. Here the bread producer enchantment dominates!

One of the main things the bread machine will do is working the batter – you will hear the sounds. On the off chance that your bread creator accompanies the preview window, you can watch the entire procedure of preparing, which is very interesting.

After the massaging stage, everything will go calm for quite a while – the rising stage comes. The machine allows the mixture to dough and rise. At that point, there will be another round of manipulating and a period of demonstrating.

At long last, the bread producer' broiler will turn on, and you will see the steam coming up through the steam vent. Although the typical bread making process is programmed, most machines accompany formula books that give you various intriguing propelled bread plans.

The best thing about using a bread-making machine is it gets the hard cycle of bread making easy. You can use the bread-making machine in complete cycle, especially for loaf bread, or you can just do the dough cycle if you are baking bread that needs to bake in an oven.

To use the bread-making machine, here are some steps to guide you:

## *Familiarize yourself with the parts and buttons of your bread-making machine.*

Your bread-making machine has three essential parts, and without it, you will not be able to cook your bread. The first part is the machine itself, the second is the bread bucket, and the third is the kneading blade. The bread bucket and kneading blade are removable and replaceable. You can check with the manufacturer for parts to replace it if it's missing.

Learn how to operate your bread-making machine. Removing and placing the bread bucket back in is important. Practice snapping the bread bucket on and off the machine until you are comfortable doing it. This is important because you don't want the bucket moving once the ingredients are in place.

## Know your bread bucket capacity.

This is an important step before you start using the machine. If you load an incorrect measurement, you are going to have a big mess on your hand. To check your bread bucket capacity:

- Use a liquid measuring cup and fill it with water.
- Pour the water on the bread bucket until it's full. Count how many cups of water you poured on the bread bucket.
- The number of cups of water will determine the size of your loaf bread
  - Less than 10 cups =1-pound loaf
  - 10 cups =1 to 1 ½ pounds loaf
  - 12 cups=1 or 1 ½ to 2 pounds loaf
  - 14 cups or more=1 or ½ to 2 or 2 ½ pounds loaf

## Learn the basic buttons and settings of your bread-making machine.

Here are some tips you can do to familiarize yourself with the machine:

- Read all the button labels. The buttons indicate the cycle in which your machine will mix, knead, and bake the bread.
- Basic buttons include START/STOP, CRUST COLOR, TIMER/ARROW, SELECT (BASIC, SWEET, WHOLE WHEAT, FRENCH, GLUTEN FREE, QUICK/RAPID, QUICK BREAD, JAM, DOUGH.)
- The SELECT button allows you to choose the cycle you want in which you want to cook your loaf. It also includes DOUGH cycle for oven-cooked breads.

## Using the Delay button.

When you select a cycle, the machine sets a preset timer to bake the bread. For example, if you select BASIC, time will be set by 3 hours. However, you want your bread cooked at a specific time, say, you want it in the afternoon, but it's only 7:00 in the morning. Your bread cooks for 3 hours, which means it will be done by 10:00 am, but you want it done by 12. You can use the up and down arrow key to set the delay timer. Between 7 am and 12 noon, there is a difference of 5 hours, so you want your timer to be set at 5. Press the arrow keys up to add 2 hours in your timer so that your bread will cook in 5 hours instead of 3 hours. Delay button does not work if you are using the DOUGH cycle.

## Order of adding the ingredients

This only matters if you are using the delay timer. It is important to ensure that your yeast will not touch any liquid so as not to activate it early. Early activation of the yeast could make your bread rise too much. If you plan to start the cycle immediately, you can add the ingredients in any order. However, adding the ingredients in order will discipline you to do it every time and make you less likely to forget it when necessary. To add the ingredients, do it in the following order:

- First, place all the liquid ingredients in the bread bucket.
- Add the sugar and the salt.
- Add the flour to cover and seal in the liquid ingredients.
- Add all the other remaining dry ingredients.
- Lastly, add the yeast. The yeast should not touch any liquid until the cooking cycle starts. When adding the yeast, make a small well using your finger to place the yeast to ensure proper timing of yeast activation.

## Using the Dough Cycle

You cannot cook all breads using the bread-making machine, but you can use the machine to make the bread-making process easier. All bread goes under the dough cycle. If your bread needs to be oven-cooked, you can still use the bread-making machine by selecting the DOUGH cycle to mix and knead your flour into a dough. To start the Dough cycle:

- Add all your bread recipe ingredients in your bread bucket.
- Select the DOUGH cycle. This usually takes between 40 to 90 minutes.
- Press the START button.
- After the cycle is complete, let your dough rest in the bread-making machine for 5 to 40 minutes.
- Take out the dough and start cutting into your desire shape.

Some machines have Pasta Dough or Cookie Dough cycle, which you can use for muffin recipes. However, if all you have is basic dough setting, you can use it for muffin recipe, but you need to stop the machine before the rising cycle begins.

## How to Use a Bread Machine?

Independent of which bread machine you pick, the preparing procedure is basically the equivalent all over the place. You load fixings to the tin. At that point, place the bread container in the machine and pick the vital program.

The average heating process takes anyplace somewhere in the range of 2 and 5 hours, contingent upon the model. Toward the finish of the heating procedure, it is prescribed to put a portion on a wire rack to chill off before eating it.

Other than the principle fixings, you can include some other additional items you need, including raisins, nuts, chocolate chips, and so forth.

While bread heating procedure may appear to be exceptionally crude and straightforward, there are a few indications that will make you a star at bread preparing with a bread machine:

Check and adhere to the guidelines/manual. With some bread creators, the dry fixings ought to be included first, with others, the wet fixings go in first.

In addition, when perusing bread preparing plans, remember that not the entirety of the bread creators is made equivalent – some item 1 pound portions, others make 1, 5, and 2 pound portions. A portion of the bread machine models is equipped for heating 3-pound portions.

It is significant not to surpass the limit of the bread machine container.

In the event that the formula calls for milk, it isn't prescribed to utilize a deferred blend cycle.

Set the machine for 'Pizza Dough' program following the manual of your bread creator. After your mixture is prepared, you can move it to a gently floured surface for additional handling.

## Benefits of a Bread Machine

While utilizing a bread machine for some may seem like a pointless advance, others don't envision the existence without newly home-heated bread. In any case, how about we go to the realities – underneath, we indicated the advantages of owning a bread machine.

As a matter of first importance, you can appreciate the crisply prepared handcrafted bread. Most bread creators additionally include a clockwork, which permits you to set the preparing cycle at a specific time. This capacity is extremely valuable when you need to have sweltering bread toward the beginning of the day for breakfast.

You can control what you eat. By preparing bread at home, you can really control what parts are coming into your portion. This choice is extremely valuable for individuals with sensitivities or for those, who attempt to control the admission of a fixings' portion.

It is simple. A few people believe that preparing bread at home is chaotic, and by and large, it is a hard procedure. In any case, preparing bread with a bread machine is a breeze. You simply pick the ideal choice and unwind - all the blending, rising, and heating process is going on within the bread producer, which additionally makes it a zero chaos process!

It sets aside you huge amounts of cash in the long haul. If you imagine that purchasing bread at a store is modest, you may be mixed up. In turns out that in the long haul, preparing bread at home will set aside your cash, particularly in the event that you have some dietary limitations.

Bread machines can create different sorts of bread: whole wheat bread, sans gluten bread, rye bread, and several different kinds. They can likewise make pizza mixture, pasta batter, jam, and different heavenly dishes.

Incredible taste and quality, you have to acknowledge it – nothing beats the quality and taste of a crisp heap of bread. Since you are the person who is making bread, you can ensure that you utilize just the fixings that are new and of a high caliber. Homemade bread consistently beats locally acquired bread as far as taste and quality.

## What Else Can you Do with a Bread Machine?

We have just referenced that bread creator utilizes are not just constrained to heating various kinds of bread. Here, we might want to investigate some inventive thoughts regarding how to utilize a bread machine.

### You Can Create Your Own Fruit or Vegetable Butters

Bread machine is an extraordinary apparatus for making creamy fruit spread. He featured that the gradual warmth inside the bread machine builds up the sugars in the organic product.

### It Is Possible to Make Delicious tomato Sauce in a Bread Maker

A bread machine is in the same class as a stewing pot. Be that as it may, it accepts that the unsettling part makes the bread machine ideal for a sauce.

### Prepare a Casserole? Of Course!

Any dish you can envision can be made in a bread creator rather than a customary stove.

### Bread Makers Can Bake Cakes

Similarly, likewise, with ideal portions of bread, bread making machines are incredible for heating cakes.

## Bread Machine Setting Programs

Most bread machines offer a number of settings. While they may be called slightly different things the most common include:

### Basic

This is the most commonly used settings. Often used for traditional white loaves. This setting is what will be used for many savory yeast recipes. This setting should not be used when making sweet bread, which can cause over proofing and will result in overflowing.

### Whole Wheat

If you are making a bread that uses whole wheat flour, then this is the setting you will use. Whole wheat flour requires a longer bake time. If you use a wheat gluten ingredient, then you may be able to use the basic setting instead. Double check your user manual to understand which settings are best based on the ingredients you are using.

### Gluten-Free

Most of the time, the flours used in these recipes act differently than the everyday all-purpose flour or even wheat flour. Many gluten-free recipes will vary slightly or significantly, but most ingredients should be set out and used at room temperature. Many of these breads, although gluten-free, will still require a rise time.

## Sweet Bread

This setting is also used often. This setting is what will be used for most sweet bread recipes that include yeast.

## French

This setting is what will be used for not just French bread, but different types of artisan breads. When using this setting, you will have a bread that comes out with a crispy crust like that of a French or Italian loaf.

## Quick/Rapid

This setting may also be labeled either quick cycle or rapid time. These breads will bake quickly and have short rise times. If using a rapid rising yeast, you can sometimes use this setting. To use this setting correctly, consult the user manual of your specific machine to ensure proper use.

## Quick Bread

This setting is used for most breads that require no rising times and can be baked immediately. Banana bread is one example of a recipe you would use this setting for. This setting can also be used to bake cakes in your bread machine as well.

## Jam

Some bread machines will offer special settings such as jam. This setting allows you to make your own homemade jams.

## Dough

This is another special setting that some bread machines may offer. The dough setting can be used to make the dough for different breads, pies crust, and even cookie dough.

# Basic Steps to Make Bread

Bread is usually prepared from combining flour and water to form a dough and commonly cooked by baking. Bread has played a significant role in the history of human-made food throughout the world.

Below is a basic guide on how to make bread:

- Scaling refers to measuring of ingredients and the most important in the bread-making process. A slight change in the measurement can affect how your bread will turn out.

- Mix all ingredients you measure to prepare it for fermentation and development of gluten. The key to mixing is time and speed.

- Next is allowing the dough to rise or the fermentation process. During this time, the yeast converts the dough's natural sugars into carbon dioxide and ethanol. The carbon dioxide is what makes the dough rise.

- After fermentation, you need to release some of the trapped carbon dioxide in the gluten. This is the punching or degassing process. This process also helps gluten to relax, distribute nutrients, and equalize the temperature of the dough inside and out.

- Next process is cutting or dividing. Dividing the dough will help you easily manage the dough during the next stages. You can cut and weigh the dough into smaller sizes.

- The next step is shaping your dough to your desired type of bread. You can shape it into a loaf, a ball, or a long torpedo.

- Next is resting or benching. You set aside your pre-shaped dough to rest and make the gluten relax. Resting time varies from a few minutes or more.

- The next process is the final shaping and panning. After resting, you can knead the dough and get it into its final shape. You can shape it into a ball, baguette, torpedo, braid, or loaf before putting it in the baking pan.

- Most breads with yeast undergo two fermentation. The first one is bulk fermentation, and the second is during proofing. During proofing, the dough can rise to its baking size.
- After proofing, the bread is ready to go into the oven to bake.
- Once baked, the bread goes on cooling racks to cool down.
- Last step is storing and packing of the bread.

## What Kinds Of Bread Machines Are There?

Lion's share of the bread-making machines will be somewhat extraordinary. This is because of the way that every variety of bread creator is intended to fill a specific need. Beneath, we will talk about the most widely recognized kinds of bread creators accessible on the advanced market.

### Vertical

The greater part of the bread machines heat portions that are situated vertically, as the bread tin is molded right now. This sort of bread machine includes just one massaging paddle.

### Even

There are likewise some bread producers that have two working oars inside the tin. These bread machines prepare level bread, much the same as the one you get from the pastry kitchen of the shop.

### Small

Little bread producers are extraordinary for the restricted kitchen space or if you don't eat a ton of bread. These little kitchen assistants don't take a significant part of the counter space and produce simply enough bread for a couple or one individual.

## Huge

Huge bread machines prove to be useful in enormous families – bread can vanish immediately when you have many individuals at the table. The large bread creators that produce 3 lb portions of bread are equipped for sustaining a major family.

## Gluten-Free

With the incredible wealth of the bread creator models available, there are unquestionably those, which are intended to provide food the requirements of smart dieting individuals.

Much the same as that, a bread machine that has a gluten setting is perfect for preparing this sort of bread.

# Choosing the Right Bread Machine

When selecting the ideal bread machine for your home, there are several factors to have in mind. These factors include:

a) The size of the bread machine pan. If you are many in your household, then a bigger bread pan is ideal for getting bread big enough to satisfy the whole group. If you are by yourself or there are only two of you, a smaller bread pan may be ideal.

b) Bread machines are different, and they come with several cycles, as well. These cycles are what determine how best the dough will be mixed and kneaded. Bread machines with fewer cycles are ideal, but it all depends on what your needs are.

c) Bread machines come in different qualities, which also dictate their prices as well. The best qualities are, of course, more expensive. Consider what your needs are and what you can afford before purchasing one.

d) Consider the timer on your machine. Some have the timer on the dough only, which lets you know when it is ready to be removed and baked in an oven. Some have it on the bake cycle when the bread is to be baked on the bread maker itself.

e) Different machines produce bread in different shapes as well. Consider the shape you want before making a purchase. It is important to note that each shape has its challenges; one example is that horizontal-shaped pans have a problem when kneading the dough. They are notorious for leaving flour in the pan's corners.

# Producers

Presently, as we have talked about the key minutes about bread creators, ample opportunity has already passed to take a gander at the organizations that produce them. While there are many bread machine makers, existent all-inclusive, we will concentrate on the most dependable and famous bread machine producers.

## Zojirushi

The Zojirushi Corporation is a Japanese organization that produces different home machines, one of Zojirushi's product offerings - bread creators. Bread machines from this maker are known for their predominant quality.

The organization maker machines in two sizes that are mirroring the clients' inclinations. The 2 – lb Bread machines are ideal for heating customarily molded 2-lb portion. The 1-lb bread machine will be a solid match for one individual or individuals who eat less bread.

Bread machines from Zojirushi are equipped for making top-notch bread, cakes, and various dishes. Zojirushi bread creators offer the accompanying cycles: entire wheat, cake, jam, custom made (the natively constructed cycle permits you to program the work, rise and prepare times for your inclinations), and mixture.

## Panasonic

We wager you previously caught wind of Panasonic – the notorious brand behind various electronic gadgets. Panasonic Corporation is likewise recently known as Matsushita Electric Industrial Co., Ltd. The organization is a Japanese worldwide gadget maker.

Panasonic bread creators are at the highest point of the value bushel, yet the cost can be clarified by various astonishing highlights that are offered by these apparatuses.

Panasonic offers five bread creators models, with one of them highlighting a programmed yeast administering framework.

## Breadman

The organization is an American brand of kitchen machines. Breadman bread producers offer the chance to prepare proficient style bread at home. The brand is known for its unrivaled quality and reliable client service.

## Breville

Breville is an Australian little home apparatuses maker, which was set up in Melbourne in 1932. The organization is demonstrated to utilize top-notch materials for their items, and it turned out to be very well known in New Zealand and the US.

## West Bend

The West Bend Company was known as a West Bend, Wisconsin organization in the period somewhere in the range of 1911 and 2001. The West Bend Company has been creating aluminum cookware and electrical apparatuses. In any case, it is likewise known for assembling stroke cycle motors, for example, detachable pontoon engines.

With the extraordinary experience despite its good faith, West Bend Company is equipped for conveying the top of the line item to the clients. The Small Kitchen Appliance Division of the West Bend is known as West Bend Housewares.

# How to Clean a Bread Maker?

There are a few straightforward advances you can follow to keep up your bread producer appropriately. Most importantly, you have to recall the accompanying guidelines for utilizing the bread machine:

- Clean your bread producer each time you use it;

- Never pour water or some other fluid straightforwardly into the bread creator, while cleaning. Just the bread tin is intended to have fluids inside;
- Make sure that the machine is unplugged and has cooled totally before playing out any upkeep or cleaning

## *Cleaning a Bread Machine*

In the event that you need to draw out the life of your bread machine, it is important to deal with the apparatus all the time. To keep your bread creator in the ideal condition, you won't have to invest a lot of energy.

## *Stage One: Remove all the Crumbs & Residue from the Bread Tin*

After you have unplugged the bread machine and it has totally chilled off, you can begin the cleaning procedure. Turn it as an afterthought over the sink, trash, or some other surface and delicately clear the pieces of remaining flour with some wipe or delicate brush.

If there is some mixture adhered to the dividers of the bread producer tin, leave it till it dries out – and afterward expel similarly as you did with the morsels. A similar procedure ought to be followed if there is some mixture of the warming component of the bread producer.

Remember that not the entirety of the removable pieces of your bread producer is dishwasher safe. Many bread machines have parts that can be washed in the dishwashing machine. In any case, it is in every case, better to double-check and read the manual to discover the similarity part.

## Stage Two: Ensure Everything Is Dry Before Using Bread Maker Again

After you wrapped up the pieces of your bread machine, ensure that every one of them is totally dry before assembling them back. There's nothing more to it! It is that straightforward - three simple strides to keeping your bread machine consistently in incredible condition.

As a little something extra, we have arranged some more tips about cleaning and support of bread creators.

On the off chance that any fluid contacted the inward surface of the bread machine, utilize a microfiber fabric to absorb the dampness. Make a point to rehash a similar procedure until there is no wet left on the warming component.

It is critical to take great consideration of the warming component of your bread machine, as this is one of the most major pieces of the apparatus. Keep the warming component clean and don't let any earth/pieces go onto it – this represents a danger of fire. To clean the warming component, utilize a delicate fabric, and expel the earth tenderly.

# CHAPTER 5: WHAT KITCHEN TOOLS DO YOU NEED?

In addition to the bread machine, which is obviously the indispensable device for preparing recipes that you will find in the next chapters, there are other tools that can make your job easier.

You probably already have many of them in your kitchen. Here are some of the most important:

## *Kitchen scale*

Every kitchen should have a scale. It is a very important tool in baking, which is a must-have. It is practically not possible to prepare some types of foods without having a kitchen scale. For baking, a scale is necessary. It is recommended to make accurate measurements when preparing bread. This is because using a cup to measure may be wrong many times. A digital scale is recommended, as it is very accurate.

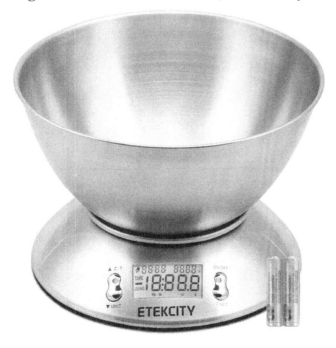

### Bowls

I love using the large metal mixing bowl that I found at a restaurant supply store, but any bowl will do. Make sure you have a variety of sizes so you can measure out different quantities of ingredients. Whenever I shop at thrift stores, I like finding small bowls for a few cents here and there to add to my collection. Having little bowls for ingredients in smaller amounts, like salt, yeast, chopped herbs, and so on, is nice, but it's not absolutely necessary—any vessel will do.

### Dough Scraper

I recommend getting metal and a plastic dough scraper. They cost just a few dollars at kitchen stores, at restaurant supply stores, or on Amazon, and they are so useful. A metal scraper is helpful for cutting and scraping dough off your work area, and a plastic scraper is flexible enough to help scrape the dough out of the bowl after rinsing.

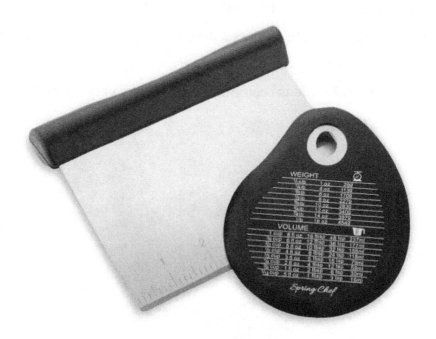

### Pastry brush

Pastry brush or basting brush looks like a paintbrush. It is made of plastic fiber or nylon. It is used for spreading butter, oil, or glaze on food.

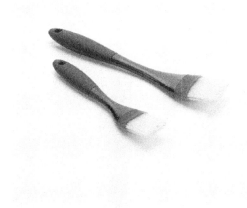

### Blender

It is an essential kitchen appliance used for emulsifying, puree, or mix food.

### Mixer

Every person needs a Mixer in their kitchen. It is a very handy kitchen tool, and it does the heaviest work – kneading the dough.

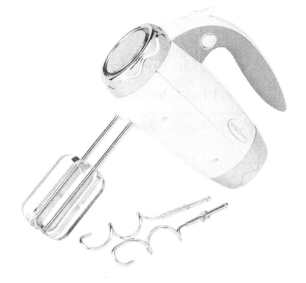

### Food processor

A food processor is good for kneading and mixing doughs, pureeing, grating cheese, or shredding and grinding items.

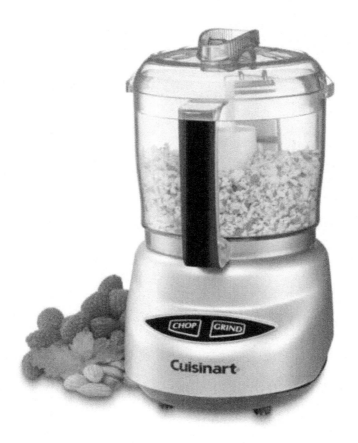

### Oven

Usually, it is essential for baking, but in this recipe book, we will only use it in some recipes because the star will be the bread machine.

### Cheese grater

Use a stainless-steel cheese grater to get your cheese perfectly grated.

## Razor Blade or Lame

A razor blade is the best tool for slashing the top of a loaf of bread. A lame is a tool that holds the razor blade safely and has a nice handle, which makes it even easier to make precision slashes.

## Rimmed Baking Sheet

This is an item you likely have in your kitchen already, and if not, it's a worthwhile investment. I usually use a 12-by-18-inch or a 16-by-24-inch baking sheet, which can be found at restaurant supply stores and online.

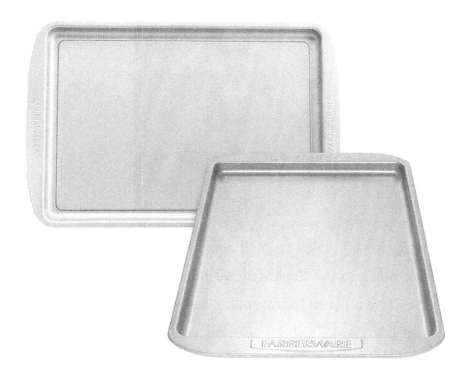

### Banneton or Proofing Basket

For the final proof, the dough needs to be placed in a basket that will allow air to circulate. You can buy baskets specifically for this called bannetons, which are made of cane. If you aren't ready to invest in a couple of bannetons just yet, a round or oval basket from a thrift store can be lined with a floured kitchen towel for a more affordable option. When I first started out, I had a ragtag collection of round and oval-shaped baskets, and they worked just fine.

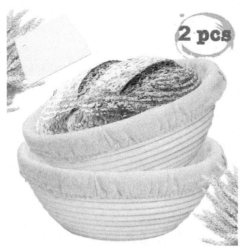

### Thermometer

To achieve consistency in your baking, you'll need to know the temperature of your water and the ingredients. Buy a probe thermometer to check temperatures of ingredients. I also recommend you have an oven thermometer to be sure the temperature of your oven is accurate. You can purchase these for around $20 on Amazon and in most grocery stores.

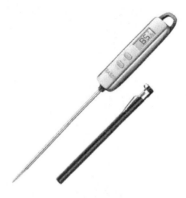

Finally, here is a small list with other useful tools that you will certainly have in the kitchen and that do not need any particular explanation:

- Kitchen towels
- Nonstick cooking spray
- Spoon
- Teaspoon
- Tablespoon
- Scissors
- Plastic wrap

# CHAPTER 6: TIPS AND FAQS FOR BREAD MACHINE BEGINNERS

## Baking Tips

Do not get frustrated if a dish does not turn out perfectly as you are baking with new ingredients, which are usually fussy and will take some practice. However, read through these tips carefully to gain the knowledge that you will require to have your Keto breads turn out to be a success!

## Temperature is everything

You want to use eggs, cream cheese, sour cream, milk and any other cooled items set at room temperature. This is due to cold items not mixing particularly well into the almond and coconut flours, which are used in Keto and if they are not brought down to room temperature, then your bread will not properly rise.

A trick for the eggs, in particular, is to use a bowl of warm water to immerse the eggs for the duration of 4 minutes. This will quickly bring them to room temperature, which is a nice trick in case you forgot to pull them out of the fridge.

Make sure that you measure your ingredients properly

This will lead to consistent results for all the Keto recipes that you find. The correct method in measuring is to spoon the ingredient into the cup rather than scooping it out of the bag directly. This will create perfect results every time as you will not over pack the ingredients using this method. You can also ensure that all the ingredients are the correct increments if you purchase a simple kitchen or baking scale.

## Ensure the yeast is properly proofed

Not every recipe includes active dry yeast. However, for the ones that do, there is a specific process to follow as outlined in those particular recipes. It includes combining the yeast with honey for the yeast to feed upon. Do not worry about the sugar content as the honey is for the yeast to feed upon, creating the carbon dioxide required for the bread to rise. The sugar will be cooked off during the process and will not be present in the final result.

Once combined, you will blend water, which is the specific temperature of 105° - 110°, which can be checked with a kitchen thermometer, or it will be slightly warm to the touch. You will know that this process was successful by the mixture becoming bubbly after waiting for a period of 7 minutes.

If there are no bubbles, simply repeat the process with the correct temperature water. You will not waste a whole dish because this occurs at the beginning of the recipe.

## Temperature is important during the rising process

You want to keep your rising bread in an environment where the temperature is not going to vary much and will be undisturbed during the rising time. You want to have the area to be slightly warm and humid, but not hot as this will stop the rising process. It is suggested to keep the covered tray on top of the stove, which is preheating.

Always Sift Your Coconut Flour:

Not sifting your coconut flour will result in a grainy bread full of coconut flour clumps...yuck! To sift your coconut flour, simply use a mesh strainer, and add the coconut flour. Sift over a large container or bowl.

## Keep away from xylitol

When using any yeast in your recipes, you want to make sure that xylitol is not an additive in your ingredients as it rapidly decreases the rising of the dough and will cause them to become flat. You will find that Monk Fruit and Erythritol do not contain xylitol and may be used as a substitute for sweeteners that have this additive included.

## Loaf pan size is important

There are a wide variety of baking pans out there. I have made it easy by including the particular pan that is required for each recipe. However, if you do not have that specific size, always opt to go with a pan that is the next size up rather than downsizing. This will ensure that the dough will not rise too far, causing the bread to burst over the pan.

The measurements for pans are calculated from the top of the pan and does not include the pan itself.

## Pure ingredients are everything

Especially when dealing with the different varieties of cheese, you want to make sure there are no preservatives or additives. Also, opt for the skim or whole milk types as these will have less water to weep during the baking process.

When baking powder is being used, it is a priority to ensure that it is as fresh as possible. Since there is no gluten present, it needs to be of the best quality to make the rising process work properly.

Not sure if your baking powder is still active? Do a small test by combining it with boiling water. If bubbles occur immediately, then your baking powder will make your bread properly rise.

# A perfect way to grease any pan

If you want to make sure that you do not run into the problem of your Keto breads sticking to the pan, this fail-proof trick will take the headache out of baking. Dissolve 2 tbps. of coconut oil in a saucepan and then apply to your pan with a pastry brush. Set in the freezer for a minimum of 20 minutes as the oil hardens. Pull out of the freezer before filling with your dough.

# Separating the eggs is a necessary step

It may seem like a pain at the time, but there is a reason that you will find the eggs are separated. This simple measure also helps the Keto breads to rise. When incorporating the whipped eggs into the batter, do not over mix. This is due to you counteracting the airiness that has been created by whipping the eggs, and your breads will not rise properly.

# Tips for Saving Time

The keto diet doesn't have to be either complicated or difficult. Although more and more keto-friendly products and food items are being made available these days, it's always better to cook your meals and bake goods at home. Though it might seem odd at the beginning, once you get the hang of things, this process will become faster, easier, and more enjoyable. Here are some time-saving tips for you:

Make riced cauliflower in bulk then use airtight containers to freeze it. That way, you can simply take the amount you need when your recipe calls for it.

For recipes that call for boiled low-carb food items, use an instant pot. This allows you to cook ingredients in bulk faster.

Stock up on parchment paper as you can use this to line your baking sheets, pans, and other similar items before placing them in the oven.

Use your freshly-baked bread loaves to make delicious sweet or savory sandwiches. Then store these in the refrigerator for meals on-the-go.

When planning which recipes to bake, check the ingredients to see if they share common items. This makes shopping a lot easier, especially if you want to make meal prepping part of your keto journey.

## Tips for Saving Money

Apart from saving time, there are also things you can do in order to save money while following the keto diet. Starting a new diet is always challenging, no matter what type of diet you choose to follow. Most of the time, you won't even know where to start. Although you've already learned all that you can about the diet, actually taking the first step towards starting it can be very intimidating.

If you want to stick with your keto journey, then you must make sure that you don't break the bank just because of it. Otherwise, you might end up deciding that the diet isn't working for you since you're losing money on it. This doesn't have to be the case! To help you out, here are some clever money-saving tips you can try:

### *Create things from scratch*

Whether you're baking pastries or cooking dishes, it's important to learn how to create things from scratch. Although it's easier and more convenient to purchase ready-made, prepackaged keto food products, doing so will surely make you lose a lot of money. If you want to stick with your budget, learning how to make homemade meals from scratch is of the essence.

### *Purchase fresh, whole ingredients*

Buying ingredients that are fresh and whole allows you to whip up healthy meals and snacks that fit right into your keto diet. In fact, a proper keto diet should be built around these types of ingredients so you can get high-quality sources of macros and the rest of the nutrients. Also, fresh and whole ingredients are a lot cheaper, which means that you can save a lot of money.

### Buy local produce, which is in season

Do research on which foods and food items are available each season. Purchasing local produce that is in season allows you to get the ingredients you need at an affordable price. As long as you know which ingredients are in season in your locale, you can start planning your meals and recipes easily and more effectively.

### Buy ingredients in bulk

Speaking of saving money on ingredients, buying in bulk also allows you to save some money. Go around your locale and check out all the food shops, supermarkets, farmer's markets, and convenience stores. That way, you can determine which places offer the freshest ingredients, which ones have the best prices, and which places offer bulk or wholesale products.

### Bake (and cook) in bulk

Of course, if you buy in bulk, it's a good idea to use these ingredients in bulk too. This is where meal prepping comes in. Once a week, set aside some time to plan your meals, shop for all of the ingredients and bake/cook all of your meals for the whole week. This is an excellent way to save money and ensure that you don't feel tempted to buy takeout or ready-made foods, which are less healthy and more expensive.

## Maintaining a Low-Carb Diet

Although starting the low-carb keto diet may help you lose weight, there are some things for you to consider. First of all, if you really want to shed those unwanted pounds and enjoy all of the health benefits the keto diet has to offer, you must follow it properly.

Also, to stay on the safe side, you may want to consult with your doctor before you start this diet. This is especially true for people who are suffering from medical conditions or for those who have a complicated medical history. If you've already decided to go low-carb, here are some pointers for you:

### *Choose your carbs wisely*

The main energy sources of the body come from simple and complex carbs. Simple carbs are naturally found in milk and fruits, but sweets such as candies also contain them. When choosing foods that contain carbs, opt for complex variety such as starchy veggies, lentils, beans, and legumes.

### *Opt for lean protein*

Just because you're allowed to eat moderate amounts of protein while on the keto diet, this doesn't mean that you should eat all kinds of protein. If you want to lose weight and improve your health, then the best protein choices are eggs, beans, skinless turkey or chicken breast, and fish.

## Make it a habit to read food labels

This allows you to choose the ingredients and food items that fit into your diet more effectively. When you read food labels, this gives you information about the food items you plan to purchase from stores.

Consume a lot of non-starchy veggies and fruits

Although these food items may contain simple carbs, that doesn't mean you should stop eating them. Fruits and veggies are the healthiest kinds of foods, so continue eating them as part of your diet to ensure your overall health.

## Plan your meals

Meal planning can be your friend when you're following the keto diet. This involves planning your meals for a specific amount of time (like for one week), shopping for ingredients, then setting one day each week to cook all of the meals you've planned. It's an excellent way to save time, money, and to stick with your diet.

# Maintain open communication with your doctor

Finally, it's important to maintain open communication with your doctor, especially when you experience any changes because of the diet. Whether you're at the peak of your health or you're suffering from any kind of medical condition, keeping your doctor in the loop is essential.

# Learn How to Check Nutritional Information

As mentioned, it's important to check food labels. In fact, you should make this a habit if you decide to start the keto diet. The good news is that all of the big food companies have introduced new nutrition labels, which makes it easier to learn the nutritional information of the foods you plan to buy. Here are some steps to follow when checking nutritional information:

## *Check the serving size*

This information tells you how many calories and nutrients you would get for each serving of the food item. When you know this, you can compare this serving size with the amount you actually consume.

## *Check the caloric information*

This information tells you the amount of energy you obtain for each serving.
Check the percent daily value
This information tells you the percentage of nutrients on a scale which, in turn, tells you if the food item contains minimal or high amounts of nutrients. A DV of 5% and below is considered little, and a DV of 15% and above is considered a lot.

## *Search for these nutrients*

Look for calcium, fiber, iron, vitamin A, and vitamin C.
Conversely, try to avoid these

### Cholesterol, fat, saturated fat, sodium, and trans fat.

The great thing about nutrition labels is these make it easier to compare products, they allow you to find out the nutritional value of food items, and they help you determine whether or not different food items are appropriate for your diet.

## FAQs

### What is the difference between a ketogenic diet and a low-carb diet?

A low carb diet is a general term used to describe any diet containing 130 to 150 grams on the total. However, ketogenic diets are a subset of this general diet plan. It further restricts the amount of carbohydrate to minimum levels and, at the same time, requires an increased intake of fat. Thus, a ketogenic diet plan is more specific than the low carbohydrate plan.

### Do I need to count calories? Are calories of importance?

Keeping track of caloric intake is important as it directly relates to weight gain. Whether on a low carb diet or a high one, it is necessary to keep check of the calories.

### How can a person track carb intake/ macro?

Whenever you follow a recipe, look for its contents and the nutritional value available with the recipe. If it is not available, look for online nutrition calculators, which enables you to calculate the nutritional value within a few minutes.

### What is the time taken to get to ketosis?

If you are a person of discipline and routine, then it typically takes two to three days to start a keto routine. However, it is a gradual process and goes through different stages. Exercise helps boosts the speed of the process. For people with sedentary lifestyles, it can also take weeks.

### Can I eat dairy?

This is perhaps the most frequently asked question by the people who are new to a keto diet. Not all dairy products are keto-friendly as raw dairy products are high in carbs. But those fermented or processed loses their carbohydrates and are good to use. These include butter, cheese and yogurt.

### Can I eat peanuts?

Not all legumes are not keto-friendly, peanuts are one of them. There is a great misconception that peanuts can be taken on a keto diet, but it is clearly not true as they are low on carbs and high in fats. When taken in small amounts, they do not disrupt the balance of the ketogenic diet.

### Is ketosis bad?

There is no proven evidence that could suggest that ketosis is dangerous. Many people confuse ketosis with ketoacidosis, the latter is a health problem which only occurs in patients with diabetes type 1. During ketoacidosis, the ketones level in the blood exceeds up to a critical value. Ketosis, on the other hand, is completely normal and doesn't pose any danger to a person's health.

### Are the high-fat foods healthy? Does eating a lot of fat make people fat?

Most of us believe that high fats are unhealthy, but it is nothing but a myth. Fats can only be unhealthy if taken with a high amount of carbohydrates. However, when taken with low carbs or no carbs, these fats become a direct and active source of energy for the body. They easily break down and release essential compounds, including ketones.

### Can I go off of the ketogenic diet plan and still keep the weight off?

Unfortunately, when you see-saw on any diet plan, you're going to gain the weight back. Some individuals don't understand that you're making a lifestyle change.

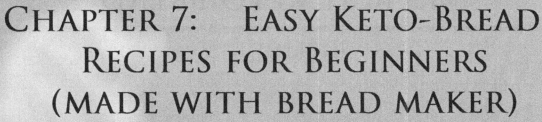

# CHAPTER 7:    EASY KETO-BREAD RECIPES FOR BEGINNERS (MADE WITH BREAD MAKER)

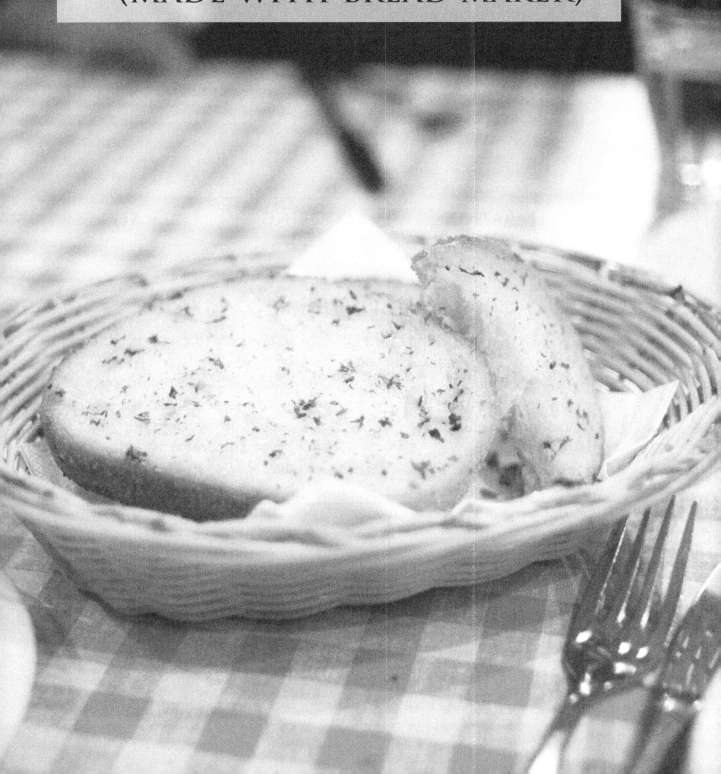

# 1. BEST KETO BREAD

## INGREDIENTS

- 1 ½ cup almond flour
- 6 drops liquid stevia
- 1 pinch Pink Himalayan salt
- ¼ tsp. cream of tartar
- 3 tsp. baking powder
- ¼ cup butter, melted
- 6 large eggs, separated

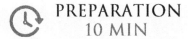 **PREPARATION** 10 MIN   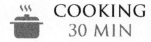 **COOKING** 30 MIN   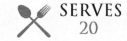 **SERVES** 20

## DIRECTIONS

1. In a bowl, to the egg whites, add cream of tartar and beat until soft peaks are formed.
2. Into another bowl, combine stevia, salt, baking powder, almond flour, melted butter. Mix well.
3. Grease the machine loaf pan with ghee.
4. Following the instructions on your machine's manual, mix the dry ingredients into the wet ingredients and pour in the bread machine loaf pan, taking care to follow how to mix in the baking powder.
5. Place the bread pan in the machine, and select the basic bread setting, together with the bread size and crust type, if available, then press start once you have closed the lid of the machine.
6. When the bread is ready, using oven mitts, remove the bread pan from the machine.
7. Let it cool before slicing.
8. Cool, slice, and enjoy.

**Nutrition:** Calories 90, Fat 7 g, Carb 2 g, Protein 3 g

# 2. YEAST BREAD

## INGREDIENTS

- 2 ¼ teaspoons dry yeast
- ½ teaspoon and 1 tablespoon erythritol sweetener, divided
- 1 1/8 cups warm water, at 100°F / 38°C
- 3 tablespoons avocado oil
- 1 cup / 100 grams almond flour
- ¼ cup / 35 grams oat fiber
- ¾ cup / 100 grams soy flour
- ½ cup / 65 grams ground flax meal
- 1 ½ teaspoons baking powder
- 1 teaspoon salt

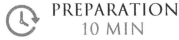 **PREPARATION**
10 MIN

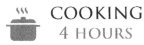 **COOKING**
4 HOURS

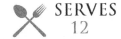 **SERVES**
12

## DIRECTIONS

1. Gather all the ingredients for the bread and plug in the bread machine having the capacity of 2 pounds of bread recipe.
2. Pour water into the bread bucket, stir in ½ teaspoon sugar and yeast and let it rest for 10 minutes until emulsified.
3. Meanwhile, take a large bowl, place the remaining ingredients in it and stir until mixed.
4. Pour flour mixture over yeast mixture in the bread bucket, shut the lid, select the "basic/white" cycle or "low-carb" setting and then press the up/down arrow button to adjust baking time according to your bread machine; it will take 3 to 4 hours.
5. Then press the crust button to select light crust if available, and press the "start/stop" button to switch on the bread machine.
6. When the bread machine beeps, open the lid, then take out the bread basket and lift out the bread.
7. Let bread cool on a wire rack for 1 hour, then cut it into twelve slices and serve.

**Nutrition:** Calories 162, Fat 11.3 g, Protein 8.1 g, Carb 7 g, Fiber 2.8 g, Net Carb 4 g

# 3. CREAM CHEESE BREAD

## INGREDIENTS

- ¼ cup / 60 grams butter, grass-fed, unsalted
- 1 cup and 3 tablespoons / 140 grams cream cheese, softened
- 4 egg yolks, pasteurized
- 1 teaspoon vanilla extract, unsweetened
- 1 teaspoon baking powder
- ¼ teaspoon of sea salt

- 2 tablespoons monk fruit powder
- ½ cup / 65 grams peanut flour

 **PREPARATION**
10 MIN

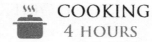 **COOKING**
4 HOURS

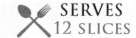 **SERVES**
12 SLICES

## DIRECTIONS

1. Gather all the ingredients for the bread and plug in the bread machine having the capacity of 2 pounds of bread recipe.

2. Take a large bowl, place butter in it, beat in cream cheese until thoroughly combined and then beat in egg yolks, vanilla, baking powder, salt, and monk fruit powder until well combined.

3. Add egg mixture into the bread bucket, top with flour, shut the lid, select the "basic/white" cycle or "low-carb" setting and then press

the up/down arrow button to adjust baking time according to your bread machine; it will take 3 to 4 hours.

4. Then press the crust button to select light crust if available, and press the "start/stop" button to switch on the bread machine.

5. When the bread machine beeps, open the lid, then take out the bread basket and lift out the bread.

6. Let bread cool on a wire rack for 1 hour, then cut it into twelve slices and serve.

**Nutrition:** Calories 98, Fat 7.9 g, Protein 3.5 g, Carb 2.6 g, Fiber 0.4 g, Net Carb 2.2 g

# 4. LEMON POPPY SEED BREAD

## INGREDIENTS

- 3 eggs, pasteurized
- 1 ½ tablespoons butter, grass-fed, unsalted, melted
- 1 ½ tablespoons lemon juice
- 1 lemon, zested
- 1 ½ cups / 150 grams almond flour
- ¼ cup / 50 grams erythritol sweetener
- ¼ teaspoon baking powder
- 1 tablespoon poppy seeds

 **PREPARATION**
10

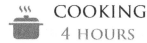 **COOKING**
4 HOURS

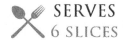 **SERVES**
6 SLICES

## DIRECTIONS

1. Gather all the ingredients for the bread and plug in the bread machine having the capacity of 1 pound of bread recipe.
2. Take a large bowl, crack eggs in it and then beat in butter, lemon juice, and lemon zest until combined.
3. Take a separate large bowl, add flour in it and then stir in sweetener, baking powder, and poppy seeds until mixed.
4. Add egg mixture into the bread bucket, top with flour mixture, shut the lid, select the "basic/white" cycle or "low-carb" setting and then press the up/down arrow button to adjust baking time according to your bread machine; it will take 3 to 4 hours.
5. Then press the crust button to select light crust if available, and press the "start/stop" button to switch on the bread machine.
6. When the bread machine beeps, open the lid, then take out the bread basket and lift out the bread.
7. Let bread cool on a wire rack for 1 hour, then cut it into six slices and serve.

**Nutrition:** Calories 201, Fat 17.5 g, Protein 8.2 g, Carb 5.8 g, Fiber 3 g, Net Carb 2.8 g

# 5. ALMOND MEAL BREAD

## INGREDIENTS

- 4 eggs, pasteurized
- ¼ cup / 60 ml melted coconut oil
- 1 tablespoon apple cider vinegar
- 2 ¼ cups / 215 grams almond meal
- 1 teaspoon baking soda
- ¼ cup / 35 grams ground flaxseed meal

- 1 teaspoon onion powder
- 1 tablespoon minced garlic
- 1 teaspoon of sea salt
- 1 teaspoon chopped sage leaves
- 1 teaspoon fresh thyme
- 1 teaspoon chopped rosemary leaves

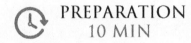 **PREPARATION** 10 MIN

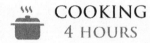 **COOKING** 4 HOURS

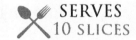 **SERVES** 10 SLICES

## DIRECTIONS

1. Gather all the ingredients for the bread and plug in the bread machine having the capacity of 2 pounds of bread recipe.
2. Take a large bowl, crack eggs in it and then beat in coconut oil and vinegar until well blended.
3. Take a separate large bowl, place the almond meal in it, add remaining ingredients, and stir until well mixed.
4. Add egg mixture into the bread bucket, top with flour mixture, shut the lid, select the "basic/white" cycle or "low-carb" setting and then press the up/down arrow button to adjust baking time according to your bread machine; it will take 3 to 4 hours.
5. Then press the crust button to select light crust if available, and press the "start/stop" button to switch on the bread machine.
6. When the bread machine beeps, open the lid, then take out the bread basket and lift out the bread.
7. Let bread cool on a wire rack for 1 hour, then cut it into ten slices and serve.

**Nutrition:** Calories 104, Fat 8.8 g, Protein 4 g, Carb 2.1 g, Fiber 1.8 g, Net Carb 0.3 g

# 6. MACADAMIA NUT BREAD

## INGREDIENTS

- 1 cup / 135 grams macadamia nuts
- 5 eggs, pasteurized
- ½ teaspoon apple cider vinegar
- ¼ cup / 30 grams coconut flour
- ½ teaspoon baking soda

 **PREPARATION** MIN      **COOKING** MIN      **SERVES** 2

## DIRECTIONS

1. Gather all the ingredients for the bread and plug in the bread machine having the capacity of 1 pound of bread recipe.
2. Place nuts in a blender, pulse for 2 to 3 minutes until mixture reaches a consistency of butter, and then blend in eggs and vinegar until smooth.
3. Stir in flour and baking soda until well mixed.
4. Add the batter into the bread bucket, shut the lid, select the "basic/white" cycle or "low-carb" setting and then press the up/down arrow button to adjust baking time according to your bread machine; it will take 3 to 4 hours.
5. Then press the crust button to select light crust if available, and press the "start/stop" button to switch on the bread machine.
6. When the bread machine beeps, open the lid, then take out the bread basket and lift out the bread.
7. Let bread cool on a wire rack for 1 hour, then cut it into eight slices and serve.

**Nutrition:** Calories 155, Fat 14.3 g, Protein 5.6 g, Carb 3.9 g, Fiber 3 g, Net Carb 0.9 g

# 7. CAULIFLOWER AND GARLIC BREAD

## INGREDIENTS

- 5 eggs, pasteurized, separated
- 2/3 cup / 85 grams coconut flour
- 1 ½ cup / 300 grams riced cauliflower
- 1 teaspoon minced garlic
- ½ teaspoon of sea salt
- ½ tablespoon chopped rosemary
- ½ tablespoon chopped parsley
- ¾ tablespoon baking powder
- 3 tablespoons melted butter, grass-fed, unsalted

 **PREPARATION** 10 MIN     **COOKING** 4HOUR     **SERVES** 9

## DIRECTIONS

1. Gather all the ingredients for the bread and plug in the bread machine having the capacity of 2 pounds of bread recipe.
2. Take a medium bowl, place cauliflower rice in it, cover with a plastic wrap, and then microwave for 3 to 4 minutes until steamed.
3. Then drain the cauliflower, wrap in cheesecloth and twist well to squeeze out moisture as much as possible, set aside until required.
4. Place egg whites in a large bowl and whisk by using an electric whisker until stiff peaks form.
5. Then transfer one-fourth of whipped egg whites into a food processor, add remaining ingredients except for cauliflower and pulse for 2 minutes until blended.
6. Add cauliflower rice, pulse for 2 minutes until well combined, and then pulse in remaining egg whites until just mixed.
7. Add batter into the bread bucket, shut the lid, select the "basic/white" cycle or "low-carb"

setting and then press the up/down arrow button to adjust baking time according to your bread machine; it will take 3 to 4 hours.

8. Then press the crust button to select light crust if available, and press the "start/stop" button to switch on the bread machine.

9. When the bread machine beeps, open the lid, then take out the bread basket and lift out the bread.

10. Let bread cool on a wire rack for 1 hour, then cut it into nine slices and serve.

**Nutrition:** Calories 108, Fat 8 g, Protein 6 g, Carb 8 g, Fiber 5 g, Net Carb 3 g

# 8. ROSEMARY BREAD

## INGREDIENTS

- 6 eggs, pasteurized
- 8 tablespoons butter, grass-fed, unsalted, melted
- ½ cup /65 grams coconut flour
- 1 teaspoon baking powder
- ¼ teaspoon salt
- ½ teaspoon onion powder
- 1 teaspoon garlic powder
- 2 teaspoons dried rosemary

 **PREPARATION** 10 MIN    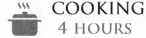 **COOKING** 4 HOURS    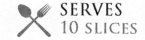 **SERVES** 10 SLICES

## DIRECTIONS

1. Gather all the ingredients for the bread and plug in the bread machine having the capacity of 1 pound of bread recipe.
2. Take a large bowl, crack eggs in it, and then slowly beat in the melted butter until well combined.
3. Take a separate large bowl, place flour in it, and then stir in remaining ingredients until mixed.
4. Add egg mixture into the bread bucket, top with flour mixture, shut the lid, select the "basic/white" cycle or "low-carb" setting and then press the up/down arrow button to adjust baking time according to your bread machine; it will take 3 to 4 hours.
5. Then press the crust button to select light crust if available, and press the "start/stop" button to switch on the bread machine.
6. When the bread machine beeps, open the lid, then take out the bread basket and lift out the bread.
7. Let bread cool on a wire rack for 1 hour, then cut it into ten slices and serve.

**Nutrition:** Calories 147, Fat 12.5 g, Protein 4.6 g, Carb 3.5 g, Fiber 2 g, Net Carb 1.5 g

# 9. SESAME AND FLAX SEED BREAD

## INGREDIENTS

- 3 eggs, pasteurized
- ½ cup / 100 grams cream cheese, softened
- 6 ½ tablespoons heavy whipping cream
- ¼ cup / 60 ml melted coconut oil
- ½ cup / 50 grams almond flour
- ¼ cup /35 grams flaxseed
- 6 ½ tablespoons coconut flour
- 2 2/3 tablespoons sesame seeds
- ½ teaspoon salt
- 1½ teaspoon baking powder
- 2 tablespoons ground psyllium husk powder
- ½ teaspoon ground caraway seeds

---

 **PREPARATION**
10 MIN

 **COOKING**
4 HOURS

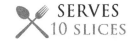 **SERVES**
10 SLICES

## DIRECTIONS

1. Gather all the ingredients for the bread and plug in the bread machine having the capacity of 2 pounds of bread recipe.
2. Take a large bowl, crack eggs in it and then beat in cream cheese, whipping cream, and coconut oil until well blended.
3. Take a separate large bowl, place flours in it, and then stir in remaining ingredients until mixed.
4. Add egg mixture into the bread bucket, top with flour mixture, shut the lid, select the "basic/white" cycle or "low-carb" setting and then press the up/down arrow button to adjust baking time according to your bread machine; it will take 3 to 4 hours.
5. Then press the crust button to select light crust if available, and press the "start/stop" button to switch on the bread machine.
6. When the bread machine beeps, open the lid, then take out the bread basket and lift out the bread.
7. Let bread cool on a wire rack for 1 hour, then cut it into ten slices and serve.

**Nutrition:** Calories 230, Fat 21 g, Protein 6.3, Carb 6.2 g, Fiber 2 g, Net Carb 3.2 g

# 10. 3-SEED BREAD

## INGREDIENTS

- 2 eggs, pasteurized
- ¼ cup / 50 grams butter melted
- 1 cup / 250 ml water warm, at 100°F / 38°C
- ¼ cup / 35 grams chia seeds
- ½ cup / 75 grams pumpkin seeds
- ½ cup / 75 grams psyllium husks
- ½ cup / 75 grams sunflower seeds
- ¼ cup / 25 grams coconut flour
- 1/4 teaspoon salt
- 1 teaspoon baking powder

 **PREPARATION** 10 MIN

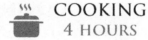 **COOKING** 4 HOURS

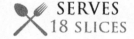 **SERVES** 18 SLICES

## DIRECTIONS

1. Gather all the ingredients for the bread and plug in the bread machine having the capacity of 2 pounds of bread recipe.
2. Take a medium bowl, crack eggs in it and then beat in the butter until well blended.
3. Take a separate large bowl, place flour in it, and then stir in remaining ingredients except for water until mixed.
4. Pour water into the bread bucket, add egg mixture, top with flour mixture, shut the lid, select the "basic/white" cycle or "low-carb" setting and then press the up/down arrow button to adjust baking time according to your bread machine; it will take 3 to 4 hours.
5. Then press the crust button to select light crust if available, and press the "start/stop" button to switch on the bread machine.
6. When the bread machine beeps, open the lid, then take out the bread basket and lift out the bread.
7. Let bread cool on a wire rack for 1 hour, then cut and serve.

**Nutrition:** Calories 139, Fat 10 g, Protein 5 g, Carb 5.6 g, Fiber 3.6 g, Net Carb 2 g

# 11. BACON AND CHEDDAR BREAD

## INGREDIENTS

- 2 eggs, pasteurized
- ¼ cup / 60 ml beer
- 2 tablespoons butter, grass-fed, unsalted, melted
- ¼ cup / 50 grams bacon, pasteurized, cooked, crumbled
- ½ cup / 120 grams shredded cheddar cheese
- ½ tablespoon coconut flour
- 1 cup / 100 grams almond flour
- ¼ teaspoon salt
- ½ tablespoon baking powder

 **PREPARATION**
10 MIN

 **COOKING**
4 HOURS

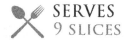 **SERVES**
9 SLICES

## DIRECTIONS

1. Gather all the ingredients for the bread and plug in the bread machine having the capacity of 2 pounds of bread recipe.
2. Take a large bowl, crack eggs in it, beat in beer and butter until blended, and then fold in bacon and cheese until just mixed.
3. Take a separate large bowl, place flours in it, and then stir in salt and baking powder until mixed.
4. Add egg mixture into the bread bucket, top with flour mixture, shut the lid, select the "basic/white" cycle or "low-carb" setting and then press the up/down arrow button to adjust baking time according to your bread machine; it will take 3 to 4 hours.
5. Then press the crust button to select light crust if available, and press the "start/stop" button to switch on the bread machine.
6. When the bread machine beeps, open the lid, then take out the bread basket and lift out the bread.
7. Let bread cool on a wire rack for 1 hour, then cut it into nine slices and serve.

**Nutrition:** Calories 140, Fat 12 g, Protein 5 g, Carb 3 g, Fiber 1 g, Net Carb 2 g

# 12. OLIVE BREAD

## INGREDIENTS

- 4 eggs, pasteurized
- 4 tablespoons avocado oil
- 1 tablespoon apple cider vinegar
- ½ cup / 65 grams coconut flour
- 1 tablespoon baking powder
- 2 tablespoons psyllium husk powder
- 1 ½ tablespoons dried rosemary
- 1/2 teaspoon salt
- 1/3 cup / 75 grams black olives, chopped
- ½ cup / 120 ml boiling water

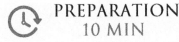 **PREPARATION** 10 MIN

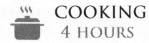 **COOKING** 4 HOURS

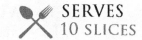 **SERVES** 10 SLICES

## DIRECTIONS

1. Gather all the ingredients for the bread and plug in the bread machine having the capacity of 2 pounds of bread recipe.
2. Take a medium bowl, crack eggs in it, blend in oil until combined, stir in vinegar and fold in olives until mixed.
3. Take a separate medium bowl, place flour in it, and then stir in husk powder, baking powder, salt, and rosemary until mixed.
4. Add egg mixture into the bread bucket, top with flour mixture, shut the lid, select the "basic/white" cycle or "low-carb" setting and then press the up/down arrow button to adjust baking time according to your bread machine; it will take 3 to 4 hours.
5. Then press the crust button to select light crust if available, and press the "start/stop" button to switch on the bread machine.
6. When the bread machine beeps, open the lid, then take out the bread basket and lift out the bread.
7. Let bread cool on a wire rack for 1 hour, then cut it into ten slices and serve.

**Nutrition:** Calories 85, Fat 6.5 g, Protein 2 g, Carb 3.4 g, Fiber 2.5 g, Net Carb 1 g

# 13. JALAPENO CHEESE BREAD

## INGREDIENTS

- 2 tablespoons Greek yogurt, full-fat
- 4 eggs, pasteurized
- 1/3 cup / 40 grams coconut flour
- ½ teaspoon of sea salt
- 2 tablespoons whole psyllium husks
- 1 teaspoon baking powder
- ¼ cup / 30 grams diced pickled jalapeños
- ¼ cup / 30 grams shredded cheddar cheese, divided

---

 **PREPARATION**
10 MIN

 **COOKING**
4 HOURS

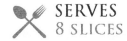 **SERVES**
8 SLICES

---

## DIRECTIONS

1. Gather all the ingredients for the bread and plug in the bread machine having the capacity of 1 pound of bread recipe.
2. Take a large bowl, add yogurt and eggs in it and then beat until well combined.
3. Take a separate bowl, place flour in it, add remaining ingredients, and stir until mixed.
4. Add egg mixture into the bread bucket, top with flour mixture, shut the lid, select the "basic/white" cycle or "low-carb" setting and then press the up/down arrow button to adjust baking time according to your bread machine; it will take 3 to 4 hours.
5. Then press the crust button to select light crust if available, and press the "start/stop" button to switch on the bread machine.
6. When the bread machine beeps, open the lid, then take out the bread basket and lift out the bread.
7. Let bread cool on a wire rack for 1 hour, then cut it into eight slices and serve.

**Nutrition:** Calories 105, Fat 6.2 g, Protein 6.6 g, Carb 3.4 g, Fiber 1.7 g, Net Carb 1.7 g

# 14. BREAD DE SOUL

## INGREDIENTS

- ¼ tsp. cream of tartar
- 2 ½ tsp. baking powder
- 1 tsp. xanthan gum
- 1/3 tsp. baking soda
- ½ tsp. salt
- 2/3 cup unflavored whey protein
- ¼ cup olive oil
- ¼ cup heavy whipping cream

- 2 drops of liquid sugar-free sweetener
- 4 eggs
- ¼ cup butter
- 12 oz. softened cream cheese

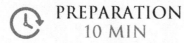 **PREPARATION** 10 MIN

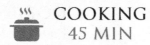 **COOKING** 45 MIN

 **SERVES** 16

## DIRECTIONS

1. Prepare bread machine loaf pan greasing it with cooking spray.
2. In a bowl, mix together the dry ingredients. Until well combined.
3. Into a separate bowl, microwave cream cheese and butter for 1 minute.
4. Remove and blend well with a hand mixer.
5. Add olive oil, eggs, heavy cream, and few drops of sweetener and blend well.
6. Following the instructions on your machine's manual, mix the dry ingredients into the wet ingredients and pour in the bread machine loaf pan, taking care to follow how to mix in the baking powder.
7. Place the bread pan in the machine, and select the basic bread setting, together with the bread size and crust type, if available, then press start once you have closed the lid of the machine.
8. When the bread is ready, using oven mitts, remove the bread pan from the machine.
9. Let it cool before slicing.
10. Cool, slice, and enjoy.

**Nutrition:** Calories 200, Fat 15.2 g, Carb 1.8 g, Protein 10 g

# 15. CHIA SEED BREAD

## INGREDIENTS

- ½ tsp. xanthan gum
- ½ cup butter
- 2 tbsp. coconut oil
- 1 tbsp. baking powder
- 1 tbsp. sesame seeds
- 1 tbsp. chia seeds
- ½ tsp. salt
- ¼ cup sunflower seeds
- 2 cups almond flour
- 7 eggs

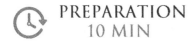 **PREPARATION** 10 MIN

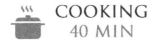 **COOKING** 40 MIN

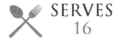 **SERVES** 16

## DIRECTIONS

1. Preheat the oven to 350F.
2. Beat eggs in a bowl on high for 1 to 2 minutes.
3. Beat in the xanthan gum and combine coconut oil and melted butter into eggs, beating continuously.
4. Set aside the sesame seeds, but add the rest of the ingredients.
5. Prepare bread machine loaf pan greasing it with cooking spray and place the mixture in it. Top the mixture with sesame seeds.
6. Place the bread pan in the machine, and select the basic bread setting, together with the bread size and crust type, if available, then press start once you have closed the lid of the machine.
7. When the bread is ready, using oven mitts, remove the bread pan from the machine.
8. Let it cool before slicing.
9. Cool, slice, and enjoy.

**Nutrition:** Calories 405, Fat 37 g, Carb 4g, Protein 14 g

# 16. SPECIAL KETO BREAD

## INGREDIENTS

- 2 tsp. baking powder
- ½ cup water
- 1 tbsp. poppy seeds
- 2 cups fine ground almond meal
- 5 large eggs
- ½ cup olive oil
- ½ tsp. fine Himalayan salt

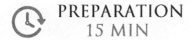 **PREPARATION** 15 MIN    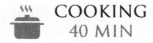 **COOKING** 40 MIN    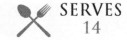 **SERVES** 14

## DIRECTIONS

1. Prepare bread machine loaf pan greasing it with cooking spray.
2. In a bowl, mix together salt, almond meal, and baking powder until well combined.
3. Following the instructions on your machine's manual, mix the dry ingredients into the wet ingredients and pour in the bread machine loaf pan, taking care to follow how to mix in the baking powder.
4. Place the bread pan in the machine, and select the basic bread setting, together with the bread size, if available, then press start once you have closed the lid of the machine.
5. When the bread is ready, using oven mitts, remove the bread pan from the machine.
6. Let it cool for 30 minutes before slicing.
7. Enjoy.

**Nutrition:** Calories 227, Fat 21 g, Carb 4 g, Protein 7 g

# 17. KETO FLUFFY CLOUD BREAD

## INGREDIENTS

- pinch salt
- ½ tbsp. ground psyllium husk powder
- ½ tbsp. baking powder
- ¼ tsp. cream of tarter
- 4 eggs, separated
- ½ cup, cream cheese

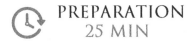 **PREPARATION** 25 MIN    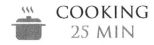 **COOKING** 25 MIN    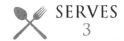 **SERVES** 3

## DIRECTIONS

1. Preheat the oven to 300F and line a baking tray with parchment paper.
2. Whisk egg whites in a bowl until soft peaks are formed.
3. Mix egg yolks with cream cheese, salt, cream of tartar, psyllium husk powder, and baking powder in a bowl.
4. Fold in the egg whites carefully and transfer to the baking tray.
5. Place in the oven and bake for 25 minutes.
6. Remove from the oven and serve.

**Nutrition:** Calories 185, Fat 16.4 g, Carb 3.9 g, Protein 6.6 g

# 18. SPLENDID LOW-CARB BREAD

## INGREDIENTS

- ½ tsp. herbs, such as basil, rosemary, or oregano
- ½ tsp. garlic or onion powder
- 1 tbsp. baking powder
- 5 tbsp. psyllium husk powder
- ½ cup almond flour
- ½ cup coconut flour
- ¼ tsp. salt
- 1 ½ cup egg whites
- 1 tbsp. oil or melted butter
- 1 tbsp. apple cider vinegar
- 1/3 to ¾ cup hot water

 **PREPARATION**
15 MIN

 **COOKING**
60-70 MIN

 **SERVES**
12

## DIRECTIONS

1. Prepare bread machine loaf pan greasing it with cooking spray.
2. In a bowl, mix together salt, psyllium husk powder, onion or garlic powder, coconut flour, almond flour, and baking powder. Until well combined.
3. Following the instructions on your machine's manual, mix the dry ingredients into the wet ingredients and pour in the bread machine loaf pan, taking care to follow how to mix in the baking powder.
4. Place the bread pan in the machine, and select the basic bread setting, together with the bread size, if available, then press start once you have closed the lid of the machine.
5. When the bread is ready, using oven mitts, remove the bread pan from the machine.
6. Cool and serve.

**Nutrition:** Calories 97, Fat 5.7 g, Carb 7.5 g, Protein 4.1 g

# 19. COCONUT FLOUR ALMOND BREAD

## INGREDIENTS

- 2 tbsp. butter, melted
- 1 tbsp. coconut oil, melted
- 6 eggs
- 1 tsp. baking soda
- 2 tbsp. ground flaxseed
- 1 ½ tbsp. psyllium husk powder
- 5 tbsp. coconut flour
- 1 ½ cup almond flour

 **PREPARATION**
10 MIN

 **COOKING**
30 MIN

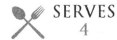 **SERVES**
4

## DIRECTIONS

1. Prepare bread machine loaf pan greasing it with cooking spray.
2. Mix the eggs in a bowl for a few minutes.
3. Add in the butter and coconut oil and mix once more for 1 minute.
4. Following the instructions on your machine's manual, add the almond flour, coconut flour, baking soda, psyllium husk, and ground flaxseed to the mixture and pour in the bread machine loaf pan.
5. Place the bread pan in the machine, and select the basic bread setting, together with the bread size, if available, then press start once you have closed the lid of the machine.
6. When the bread is ready, using oven mitts, remove the bread pan from the machine.
7. Cool and serve.

**Nutrition:** Calories 475, Fat 38 g, Carb 7 g, Protein 19 g

# 20. QUICK LOW-CARB BREAD LOAF

## INGREDIENTS

- 2/3 cup coconut flour
- ½ cup butter, melted
- 3 tbsp. coconut oil, melted
- 1/3 cup almond flour
- ½ tsp. xanthan gum
- 1 tsp. baking powder
- 6 large eggs
- ½ tsp. salt

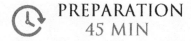 **PREPARATION**
45 MIN

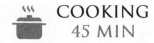 **COOKING**
45 MIN

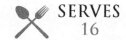 **SERVES**
16

## DIRECTIONS

1. Prepare bread machine loaf pan greasing it with cooking spray.
2. Beat the eggs until creamy.
3. Add in the coconut flour and almond flour, mixing them for 1 minute. Next, add the xanthan gum, coconut oil, baking powder, butter, and salt and mix them until the dough turns thick.
4. Pour mixture in the bread machine loaf pan.
5. Place the bread pan in the machine, and select the basic bread setting, together with the bread size, if available, then press start once you have closed the lid of the machine.
6. When the bread is ready, using oven mitts, remove the bread pan from the machine.
7. Cool and serve.

**Nutrition:** Calories 174, Fat 15 g, Carb 5 g, Protein 5 g

# 21. KETO BAKERS BREAD

## INGREDIENTS

- Pinch of salt
- 4 tbsp. light cream cheese softened
- ½ tsp. cream of tartar
- 4 eggs, yolks, and whites separated

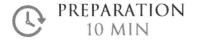
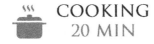
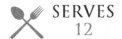

**PREPARATION**
10 MIN

**COOKING**
20 MIN

**SERVES**
12

## DIRECTIONS

1. Heat 2 racks in the middle of the oven at 350F.
2. Line 2 baking pan with parchment paper, then grease with cooking spray.
3. Separate egg yolks from the whites and place them in separate mixing bowls.
4. Beat the egg whites and cream of tartar with a hand mixer until stiff, about 3 to 5 minutes. Do not over-beat.
5. Whisk the cream cheese, salt, and egg yolks until smooth.
6. Slowly fold the cheese mix into the whites until fluffy.
7. Spoon ¼ cup measure of the batter onto the baking sheets, 6 mounds on each sheet.
8. Bake in the oven for 20 to 22 minutes, alternating racks halfway through.
9. Cool and serve.

**Nutrition:** Calories 41, Fat 3.2 g, Carb 1 g, Protein 2.4 g

# 22. ALMOND FLOUR LEMON BREAD

## INGREDIENTS

- 1 tsp. French herbs
- 1 tsp. lemon juice
- 1 tsp. salt
- 1 tsp. cream of tartar
- 1 tsp. baking powder
- ¼ cup melted butter
- 5 large eggs, divided
- ¼ cup coconut flour
- 1 ½ cup almond flour

 **PREPARATION** 15 MIN     **COOKING** 45 MIN    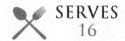 **SERVES** 16

## DIRECTIONS

1. Prepare bread machine loaf pan greasing it with cooking spray.
2. Whip the whites and cream of tartar until soft peaks form.
3. In a bowl, combine salt, egg yolks, melted butter, and lemon juice. Mix well.
4. Add coconut flour, almond flour, herbs, and baking powder. Mix well.
5. To the dough, add 1/3 the egg whites and mix until well-combined.
6. Add the remaining egg whites mixture and slowly mix to incorporate everything. Do not over mix.
7. However, take a look to the manufacturer's instructions for mixing dry and wet ingredients.
8. Pour mixture in the bread machine loaf pan.
9. Place the bread pan in the machine, and select the basic bread setting, together with the bread size, if available, then press start once you have closed the lid of the machine.

**Nutrition:** Calories 115, Fat 9.9 g, Carb 3.3 g, Protein 5.2 g

# 23. SEED AND NUT BREAD

## INGREDIENTS

- 3 eggs
- ¼ cup avocado oil
- 5 tsp. psyllium husk powder
- 1 tsp. apple cider vinegar
- ¾ tsp. salt
- 5 drops liquid stevia
- 1 ½ cups raw unsalted almonds
- ½ cup raw unsalted pepitas
- ½ cup raw unsalted sunflower seeds
- ½ cup flaxseeds

 **PREPARATION**
10 MIN

 **COOKING**
40 MIN

 **SERVES**
24

## DIRECTIONS

1. Prepare bread machine loaf pan greasing it with cooking spray.
2. In a large bowl, whisk together the oil, eggs, psyllium husk powder, vinegar, salt, and liquid stevia.
3. Stir in the pepitas, almonds, sunflower seeds, and flaxseeds until well combined.
4. However, take a look to the manufacturer's instructions for mixing dry and wet ingredients.
5. Pour mixture in the bread machine loaf pan.
6. Place the bread pan in the machine, and select the basic bread setting, together with the bread size, if available, then press start once you have closed the lid of the machine.
7. When the bread is ready, using oven mitts, remove the bread pan from the machine.
8. Cool, slice, and serve.

**Nutrition:** Calories 131, Fat 12 g, Carb 4 g, Protein 5 g

# 24. DILL AND CHEDDAR BREAD

## INGREDIENTS

- 4 eggs, pasteurized
- ¼ teaspoon cream of tartar
- 5 tablespoons butter, grass-fed, unsalted
- 2 cups / 470 grams grated cheddar cheese,
- 1 ½ cups / 150 grams almond flour
- 1 scoop of egg white protein
- 1/4 teaspoon salt
- 1 teaspoon garlic powder
- 4 teaspoons baking powder
- ¼ tablespoon dried dill weed

 **PREPARATION**
10 MIN

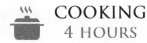 **COOKING**
4 HOURS

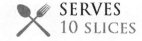 **SERVES**
10 SLICES

## DIRECTIONS

1. Gather all the ingredients for the bread and plug in the bread machine having the capacity of 2 pounds of bread recipe.
2. Take a large bowl, crack eggs in it, beat until blended and then beat in cream of tartar, butter, and cheese until just mixed.
3. Take a separate large bowl, place flour in it, and then stir in egg white protein, salt, garlic powder, baking powder, and dill until mixed.
4. Add egg mixture into the bread bucket, top with flour mixture, shut the lid, select the "basic/white" cycle or "low-carb" setting and then press the up/down arrow button to adjust baking time according to your bread machine; it will take 3 to 4 hours.
5. Then press the crust button to select light crust if available, and press the "start/stop" button to switch on the bread machine.
6. When the bread machine beeps, open the lid, then take out the bread basket and lift out the bread.
7. Let bread cool on a wire rack for 1 hour, then cut it and serve.

**Nutrition:** Calories 292, Fat 25.2 g, Protein 14.3 g, Carb 6.1 g, Fiber 2.6 g, Net Carb 3.5 g

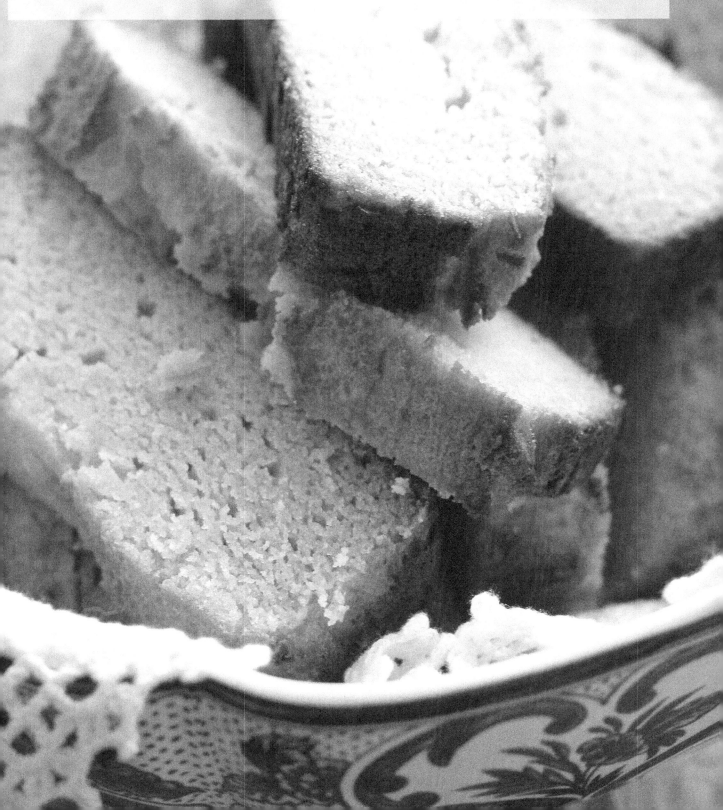

# CHAPTER 8:   GLUTEN FREE BREAD RECIPES

# 25. CLASSIC GLUTEN FREE BREAD

## INGREDIENTS

- 1/2 cup butter, melted
- 3 tbsp coconut oil, melted
- 6 eggs
- 2/3 cup sesame seed flour
- 1/3 cup coconut flour
- 2 tsp baking powder
- 1 tsp psyllium husks
- 1/2 tsp xanthan gum
- 1/2 tsp salt

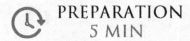 **PREPARATION** 5 MIN    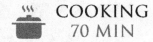 **COOKING** 70 MIN    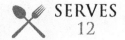 **SERVES** 12

## DIRECTIONS

1. Pour in eggs, melted butter, and melted coconut oil into your bread machine pan.
2. Add the remaining Ingredients to the bread machine pan.
3. Set bread machine to gluten free.
4. When the bread is done, remove bread machine pan from the bread machine.
5. Let cool slightly before transferring to a cooling rack.
6. You can store your bread for up to 3 days.

**Nutrition:** Calories 146, Carbohydrates 1.2 g, Protein 3.5 g, Fat 14 g

# 26. GLUTEN FREE CHOCOLATE ZUCCHINI BREAD

## INGREDIENTS

- 1 ½ cups coconut flour
- ¼ cup unsweetened cocoa powder
- ½ cup erythritol
- ½ tsp cinnamon
- 1 tsp baking soda
- 1 tsp baking powder
- ¼ tsp salt
- ¼ cup coconut oil, melted
- 4 eggs
- 1 tsp vanilla
- 2 cups zucchini, shredded

 **PREPARATION** 5 MIN      **COOKING** 80 MIN      **SERVES** 12

## DIRECTIONS

1. Shred the zucchini and use paper towels to drain excess water, set aside.
2. Lightly beat eggs with coconut oil then add to bread machine pan.
3. Add the remaining Ingredients to the pan.
4. Set bread machine to gluten free.
5. When the bread is done, remove bread machine pan from the bread machine.
6. Let cool slightly before transferring to a cooling rack.
7. You can store your bread for up to 5 days.

**Nutrition:** Calories 185, Carbohydrates 6 g, Protein 5 g, Fat 17 g

# 27. NOT YOUR EVERYDAY BREAD

## INGREDIENTS

- 2 tsp active dry yeast
- 2 tbsp inulin
- ½ cup warm water
- ¾ cup almond flour
- ¼ cup golden flaxseed, ground
- 2 tbsp whey protein isolate
- 2 tbsp psyllium husk finely ground
- 2 tsp xanthan gum
- 2 tsp baking powder
- 1 tsp salt
- ¼ tsp cream of tartar
- ¼ tsp ginger, ground
- 1 egg
- 3 egg whites
- 2 tbsp ghee
- 1 tbsp apple cider vinegar
- ¼ cup sour cream

 **PREPARATION** 5 MIN

 **COOKING** 30 MIN

 **SERVES** 12

## DIRECTIONS

1. Pour wet Ingredients into bread machine pan.
2. Add dry Ingredients, with the yeast on top.
3. Set bread machine to basic bread setting.
4. When the bread is done, remove bread machine pan from the bread machine.
5. Let cool slightly before transferring to a cooling rack.
6. You can store your bread for up to 5 days.

**Nutrition:** Calories 175, Carbohydrates 6 g, Protein 5 g, Fat 14 g

# 28. BANANA CAKE LOAF

## INGREDIENTS

- 1 ½ cups almond flour
- 1 tsp baking powder
- ½ cup butter
- 1 ½ cups erythritol
- 2 eggs
- 2 bananas, extra ripe, mashed
- 2 tsp whole almond milk

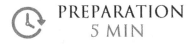 **PREPARATION**
5 MIN

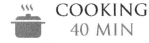 **COOKING**
40 MIN

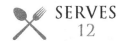 **SERVES**
12

## DIRECTIONS

1. Mix butter, eggs, and almond milk together in a mixing bowl.
2. Mash bananas with a fork and add in the mashed bananas.
3. Mix all dry Ingredients together in a separate small bowl.
4. Slowly combine dry Ingredients with wet Ingredients.
5. Pour mixture into bread machine pan.
6. Set bread machine for bake.
7. When the cake is done remove from bread machine and transfer to a cooling rack.
8. Allow to cool completely before serving.
9. You can store your banana cake loaf bread for up to 5 days in the refrigerator.

**Nutrition:** Calories 168, Carbohydrates 7 g, Protein 5 g, Fat 14 g

# 29. ALMOND BUTTER BROWNIES

## INGREDIENTS

- 1 cup almond butter
- 2 tbsp cocoa powder, unsweetened
- ½ cup erythritol
- ¼ cup dark chocolate chips, sugar-free
- 1 egg
- 3 tbsp almond milk, unsweetened

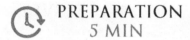 **PREPARATION** 5 MIN    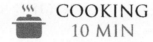 **COOKING** 10 MIN    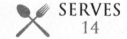 **SERVES** 14

## DIRECTIONS

1. Beat egg and almond butter together in a mixing bowl.
2. Add in erythritol and cocoa powder.
3. If the mixture is too crumbly or dry, add in almond milk until you have a smooth consistency.
4. Fold in dark chocolate chips.
5. Pour mixture into bread machine pan.
6. Set bread machine to bake.
7. When done remove from bread machine and transfer to a cooling rack.
8. Cool completely before serving, you can store for up to 5 days in the refrigerator.

**Nutrition:** Calories 141, Carbohydrates 3 g, Protein 5 g, Fat 12 g

# 30. ALMOND BUTTER BREAD

## INGREDIENTS

- 1 cup coconut almond butter, creamy
- 3 eggs
- ½ tsp baking soda
- 1 tbsp apple cider vinegar

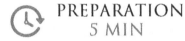 **PREPARATION** 5 MIN  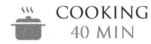 **COOKING** 40 MIN  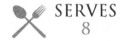 **SERVES** 8

## DIRECTIONS

1. Combine all Ingredients in a food processor.
2. When the mixture is smooth transfer to bread machine baking pan.
3. Set bread machine to bake.
4. When done baking, remove from the pan from your bread machine.
5. Allow to cool completely before slicing.
6. You can store for up to 5 days in the refrigerator.

**Nutrition:** Calories 175, Carbohydrates 6 g, Protein 5 g, Fat 14 g

# 31. GLUTEN-FREE ALMOND BREAD

## INGREDIENTS

- 2 cups almond flour, blanched
- ½ cup butter, melted
- 7 eggs
- 2 tbsp. avocado oil
- ½ tsp. xanthan gum
- ½ tsp. baking powder
- ½ tsp. salt

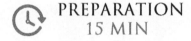 **PREPARATION** 15 MIN     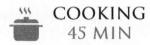 **COOKING** 45 MIN     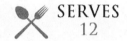 **SERVES** 12

## DIRECTIONS

1. Prepare bread machine loaf pan greasing it with cooking spray.
2. In a bowl, mix together dry Ingredients until well combined.
3. In another bowl whisk eggs for 3 minutes or until they reach a creamy consistency.
4. Following the instructions on your machine's manual, mix the dry ingredients into the wet ingredients and pour in the bread machine loaf pan, taking care to follow how to mix in the baking powder.
5. Place the bread pan in the machine, and select the basic bread setting, or gluten-free program, if available, then press start once you have closed the lid of the machine.
6. When the bread is ready, using oven mitts, remove the bread pan from the machine.
7. Let it cool before slicing.
8. Cool, slice, and serve.

**Nutrition:** Calories 247, Fat 22.8 g, Carb 4.9 g, Protein 7.7 g

# 32. KETO ALMOND BREAD

## INGREDIENTS

- ½ cups almond flour
- 2 tsp. baking powder
- 2 tbsp. butter, melted
- ¼ tsp. cream of tartar
- 6 eggs, whites and yolks separated
- Pinch of salt

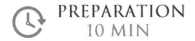 **PREPARATION** 10 MIN

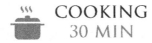 **COOKING** 30 MIN

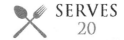 **SERVES** 20

## DIRECTIONS

1. In a bowl, beat the cream of tartar and egg whites until soft peaks form.
2. Keep the mix on the side.
3. In a food processor, mix almond flour, salt, baking powder, egg yolks, and butter.
4. Add 1/3 cup egg whites to food processor and pulse until combined.
5. Add rest of the egg whites and mix until combined.
6. Pour mixture into bread machine pan.
7. Set bread Basic program and start.
8. When baking is complete remove from bread machine and transfer to a cooling rack.
9. When it is cool, slice, and serve.

**Nutrition:** Calories 271, Fat 22 g, Carb 6 g, Protein 5 g

# 33. CARROT CAKE

## INGREDIENTS

- ½ cup erythritol
- ½ cup butter
- ½ tbsp vanilla extract
- 1 ¾ cups almond flour
- 1 ½ tsp baking powder
- 1 ½ tsp cinnamon
- ¼ tsp sea salt
- 1 ½ cup carrots, grated
- 1 cup pecans, chopped

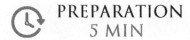 **PREPARATION**
5 MIN

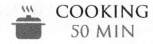 **COOKING**
50 MIN

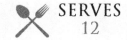 **SERVES**
12

## DIRECTIONS

1. Grate carrots and place in a food processor.
2. Add in the rest of the Ingredients, except the pecans, and process until well-incorporated.
3. Fold in pecans.
4. Pour mixture into bread machine pan.
5. Set bread machine to bake.
6. When baking is complete remove from bread machine and transfer to a cooling rack.
7. Allow to cool completely before slicing. (you can also top with a sugar-free cream cheese frosting, see recipe below).
8. You can store for up to 5 days in the refrigerator.

**Nutrition:** Calories 350, Carbohydrates 8 g, Protein 7 g, Fat 34 g

# 34. SEEDED LOAF

## INGREDIENTS

- 7 eggs
- 1 cup almond flour
- ½ cup butter
- 2 tbsp olive oil
- 2 tbsp chia seeds
- 2 tbsp sesame seeds
- 1 tsp baking soda
- ½ tsp xanthan gum
- ¼ tsp salt

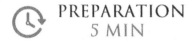 **PREPARATION** 5 MIN    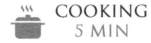 **COOKING** 5 MIN    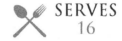 **SERVES** 16

## DIRECTIONS

1. Add eggs and butter to the bread machine pan.
2. Top with all other Ingredients.
3. Set bread machine to the gluten free setting.
4. Once done remove from bread machine and transfer to a cooling rack.
5. This bread can be stored in the fridge for up to 5 days or 3 weeks in the freezer.

**Nutrition:** Calories 190, Carbohydrates 8 g, Fats 18 g, Protein 18 g

# 35. SIMPLE KETO BREAD

## INGREDIENTS

- 3 cups almond flour
- 2 tbsp inulin
- 1 tbsp whole milk
- ½ tsp salt
- 2 tsp active yeast
- 1 ¼ cups warm water
- 1 tbsp olive oil

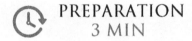 **PREPARATION**
3 MIN

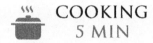 **COOKING**
5 MIN

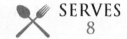 **SERVES**
8

## DIRECTIONS

1. Use a small mixing bowl to combine all dry Ingredients, except for the yeast.
2. In the bread machine pan add all wet Ingredients.
3. Add all of your dry Ingredients, from the small mixing bowl, in the bread machine pan. Top with the yeast.
4. Set the bread machine to the basic bread setting.
5. When the bread is done, remove bread machine pan from the bread machine.
6. Let cool slightly before transferring to a cooling rack.
7. The bread can be stored for up to 5 days on the counter and for up to 3 months in the freezer.

**Nutrition:** Calories 85, Carbohydrates 4 g, Fats 7 g, Protein 3 g

# 36. CLASSIC KETO BREAD

## INGREDIENTS

- 7 eggs
- ½ cup ghee
- 2 cups almond flour
- 1 tbsp baking powder
- ¼ tsp salt

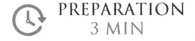 **PREPARATION**
3 MIN

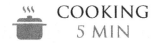 **COOKING**
5 MIN

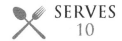 **SERVES**
10

## DIRECTIONS

1. Pour eggs and ghee into bread machine pan.
2. Add remaining Ingredients.
3. Set bread machine to quick setting.
4. Allow bread machine to complete its cycle.
5. When the bread is done, remove bread machine pan from the bread machine.
6. Let cool slightly before transferring to a cooling rack.
7. The bread can be stored for up to 4 days on the counter and for up to 3 months in the freezer.

**Nutrition:** Calories 167, Carbohydrates 2 g, Fats 16 g, Protein 5 g

# CHAPTER 9: CHEESE BREAD RECIPES

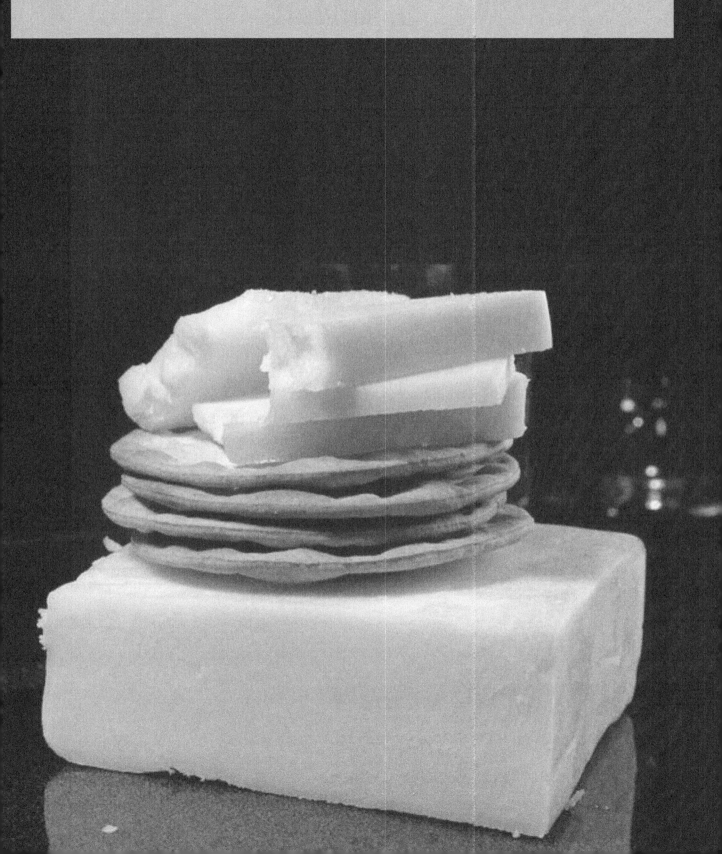

# 37. CHEESY GARLIC BREAD

## INGREDIENTS

**For Bread:**
- ¾ cup mozzarella, shredded
- ½ cup almond flour
- Salt, to taste
- 1 egg

**For topping:**
- 2 tbsp melted butter
- ½ tsp parsley
- 1 tsp garlic clove, minced

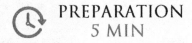 **PREPARATION**
5 MIN

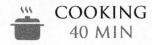 **COOKING**
40 MIN

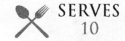 **SERVES**
10

## DIRECTIONS

1. Mix together your topping Ingredients and set aside.
2. Pour the remaining wet Ingredients into the bread machine pan.
3. Add the dry Ingredients.
4. Set bread machine to the gluten free setting.
5. When the bread is done, remove bread machine pan from the bread machine.
6. Let cool slightly before transferring to a cooling rack.
7. Once on a cooling rack, drizzle with the topping mix.
8. You can store your bread for up to 7 days.

**Nutrition:** Calories 29, Carbohydrates 1 g, Protein 2 g, Fat 2 g

# 38. CHEESY GARLIC BREAD (VERS. 2)

## INGREDIENTS

**For the Bread:**
- 5 eggs, pasteurized
- 2 cups / 200 grams almond flour
- ½ teaspoon xanthan gum
- 1 teaspoon garlic powder
- 1 teaspoon salt
- 1 teaspoon parsley
- 1 teaspoon Italian seasoning
- 1 teaspoon dried oregano
- 1 stick of butter, grass-fed, unsalted, melted

- 1 cup / 100 grams grated mozzarella cheese
- 2 tablespoons ricotta cheese
- 1 cup / 235 grams grated cheddar cheese
- 1/3 cup / 30 grams grated parmesan cheese

**For the Topping:**
- ½ stick of butter, grass-fed, unsalted, melted
- 1 teaspoon garlic powder

 **PREPARATION**
10 MIN

 **COOKING**
4 HOURS

 **SERVES**
16

## DIRECTIONS

1. Gather all the ingredients for the bread and plug in the bread machine having the capacity of 2 pounds of bread recipe.
2. Take a large bowl, crack eggs in it and then whisk until blended.
3. Take a separate large bowl, place flour in it, and stir in xanthan gum and all the cheeses until well combined.
4. Take a medium bowl, place butter in it, add all the seasonings in it, and stir until mixed.
5. Add egg mixture into the bread bucket, top with seasoning mixture and flour mixture, shut the lid, select the "basic/white" cycle or "low-carb" setting and then press the up/down arrow button to adjust baking time according to your bread machine; it will take 3 to 4 hours.
6. Then press the crust button to select light crust if available, and press the "start/stop" button to switch on the bread machine.
7. When the bread machine beeps, open the lid, then take out the bread basket and lift out the bread.
8. Prepare the topping by mixing together melted butter and garlic

powder and brush the mixture on top of the bread.

9. Let bread cool on a wire rack for 1 hour, then cut it into sixteen slices and serve.

**Nutrition:** Calories 250, Fat 14.5 g, Protein 7.2 g, Carb 3 g, Fiber 1.6 g, Net Carb 1.4 g

# 39. CHEESE BLEND BREAD

## INGREDIENTS

- 5 oz cream cheese
- 2 tsp baking powder
- ½ tsp himalayan salt
- ½ cup parmesan cheese, shredded
- 3 tbsp water
- 3 eggs
- ½ cup mozzarella cheese, shredded

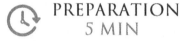 **PREPARATION 5 MIN**  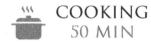 **COOKING 50 MIN**  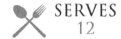 **SERVES 12**

## DIRECTIONS

1. Place wet Ingredients into bread machine pan.
2. Add dry Ingredients.
3. Set the bread machine to the gluten free setting.
4. When the bread is done, remove bread machine pan from the bread machine.
5. Let cool slightly before transferring to a cooling rack.
6. You can store your bread for up to 5 days.

**Nutrition:** Calories 132, Carbohydrates 4 g, Protein 6 g, Fat 8 g

# 40. CHEESY VEG TORTILLAS

## INGREDIENTS

- 1 ½ cups riced cauliflower
- 100g shredded cheddar cheese
- 2 free range eggs
- ½ teaspoon sea salt
- ¼ teaspoon garlic powder
- ¼ teaspoon onion powder

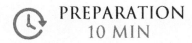 **PREPARATION** 10 MIN    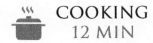 **COOKING** 12 MIN    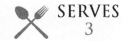 **SERVES** 3

## DIRECTIONS

1. Preheat your oven to 400 degrees f. Line three baking sheets with parchment paper and set aside.
2. Combine all Ingredients in a food processor and puree until all the Ingredients come together into a smooth texture.
3. Pour mixture in bread machine pan.
4. Place the bread pan in the machine, and select the pasta or cookies setting.
5. Then press start once you have closed the lid of the machine.
6. Remove dough from bread machine when cycle is complete.
7. Use a 3-tablespoon cookie scoop to portion the mixture onto the baking sheets, leaving room for rolling them out.
8. Cover the mounds with a piece of parchment paper. Roll the mounds out into circles until they are about 4-to 4 1/2-inches across. Remove the wax paper.
9. Bake the tortillas for 12 minutes, until golden. Cool on the baking sheets for 3-5 minutes before peeling off the parchment paper.

**Nutrition:** Calories 160, Fat 11 g, Carb 4 g, Dietary Fiber 8 g, Protein 9 g, Cholesterol 100 mg, Sodium 419 mg

# 41. CHEESE & FRUIT STUFFED PANINI

## INGREDIENTS

- Low carb flat bread (10 slices)
- 2 tbsp. Dijon mustard
- 2 tbsp. Mayonnaise
- 250g aged ham
- 120g brie thinly sliced
- 1 green apple very thinly sliced
- Oil or melted butter for brushing

 **PREPARATION**
10 MIN

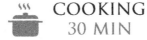 **COOKING**
30 MIN

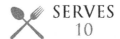 **SERVES**
10

## DIRECTIONS

1. Start by preheating your panini maker.
2. Cut through the center of each slice of bread to get two very flat and thin slices.
3. Combine mustard and mayonnaise in a small bowl and spread one side of all the slices with the combo.
4. Form sandwiches with the cheese and ham.
5. Brush the outer parts of the sandwiches with the melted butter and put in the panini maker leaving it grill until golden.

**Nutrition:** Calories 288, Total Fat 12 g, Carb 15.5 g, Dietary Fiber 7.1 g, Protein 13.6 g, Cholesterol 217 mg, Sodium 329 mg

# 42. CHEESY LOW CARB BUTTER & GARLIC BREAD

## INGREDIENTS

**For Bread:**
- 4 tablespoons melted butter
- 5 eggs
- 2 tablespoons ricotta cheese
- 1 cup mozzarella cheese
- 1 cup cheddar cheese
- 1/3 cup parmesan cheese
- 2 cups almond flour
- 1/2 teaspoon xanthan gum
- 1 teaspoon italian seasoning

- 1 teaspoon garlic powder
- 1 teaspoon oregano
- 1 teaspoon parsley
- 1 teaspoon salt

**For garlic butter spread:**
- 1 teaspoon garlic powder
- 2 tablespoons melted butter

 **PREPARATION** 5 MIN    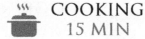 **COOKING** 15 MIN    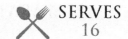 **SERVES** 16

## DIRECTIONS

1. Prepare bread machine loaf pan greasing it with cooking spray.
2. In a bowl, mix together dry Ingredients until well combined.
3. In another bowl, whisk together wet Ingredients until well blended
4. Following the instructions on your machine's manual, mix the dry ingredients into the wet ingredients and pour in the bread machine loaf pan, taking care to follow how to mix in the baking powder.
5. Place the bread pan in the machine, and select the basic bread setting, together with the bread size and crust type, if available, then press start once you have closed the lid of the machine.
6. When the bread is ready, using oven mitts, remove the bread pan from the machine.
7. Let it cool before slicing.
8. In a small bowl, whisk together melted butter and garlic until well blended. Brush with garlic butter and serve.

**Nutrition:** Calories 240, Total Fat 14 g, Carb 4 g, Dietary Fiber 1.5 g, Sugars 1 g, Protein 7 g, Cholesterol 286 mg, Sodium 302 mg

# 43. GOAT CHEESE BREAD

## INGREDIENTS

- 1 cup of almond blanched fine flour
- ½ cup of soy flour
- ¼ of salt
- 2 tsp. Of fresh thyme, crushed
- ½ cup of coconut milk, melted
- 1 tsp. Of pepper cayenne
- 2 Eggs
- 1 teaspoon Mustard of dijon
- 1 cup Crumbled fresh goat cheese
- 1 teaspoon baking powder
- 1/3 olive oil, extra virgin
- 1 teaspoon active dry yeast

 **PREPARATION** 5 MIN          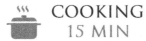 **COOKING** 15 MIN          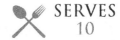 **SERVES** 10

## DIRECTIONS

1. Get a mixing container and combine the almond flour, soy flour, fresh thyme, cayenne pepper, salt, crumbled fresh goat cheese, and baking powder.
2. Get another mixing container and combine extra virgin olive oil, eggs, coconut milk, and dijon mustard.
3. As per the instructions on the manual of your machine, pour the ingredients in the bread pan, taking care to follow how to mix in the yeast.
4. Place the bread pan in the machine, and select the basic bread setting, together with the bread size and crust type, if available, then press start once you have closed the lid of the machine.
5. When the bread is ready, using oven mitts, remove the bread pan from the machine. Use a stainless spatula to extract the bread from the pan and turn the pan upside down on a metallic rack where the bread will cool off before slicing it.

**Nutrition:** Calories 134, Fat 6.8 g, Carb 4.2 g, Protein 12.1 g

# 44. RICOTTA CHIVE BREAD

## INGREDIENTS

- 1 cup lukewarm water
- 1/3 cup whole or part-skim ricotta cheese
- 1 ½ tsp salt
- 1 tablespoon granulated sugar (needed to activate yeast)
- 3 cups almond flour
- ½ cup chopped chives
- 2 ½ tsp instant yeast

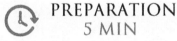 **PREPARATION** 5 MIN

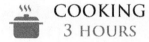 **COOKING** 3 HOURS

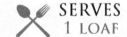 **SERVES** 1 LOAF

## DIRECTIONS

1. Add ingredients to bread machine pan except dried fruit following order in your bread machine's manual instructions, taking care on how to mix in the yeast.

2. Place the bread pan in the machine, and select the basic bread setting, together with the bread size and light/medium crust type, if available, then press start once you have closed the lid of the machine.

3. When the bread is ready, using oven mitts, remove the bread pan from the machine.

4. Use a stainless spatula to extract the bread from the pan and turn the pan upside down on a metallic rack where the bread will cool off before slicing it.

**NOTE:** Top with spreads and greens for tea time snacks.

**Nutrition:** Calories 145, Fat 18 g, Sodium 207 mg, Carb 4 g, Fiber 1 g, Protein 8 g

# 45. MOZZARELLA HERBS BREAD

## INGREDIENTS

- 1 cup grated cheese mozzarella
- ½ cup grated cheese parmesan
- ½ teaspoon salt
- 1 teaspoon baking powder
- 1 cup almond flour
- 1 cup coconut flour
- ½ cup warm water
- 1 teaspoon stevia
- ¼ teaspoon dried thyme
- 1 teaspoon grounded garlic
- 1 teaspoon dried basil

- 1 teaspoon olive oil extra virgin
- 2 teaspoons unsalted melted butter
- 1/3 cup unsweetened almond milk

 **PREPARATION** 5 MIN      **COOKING** 15 MIN      **SERVES** 10

## DIRECTIONS

1. In a mixing container, mix the almond flour, baking powder, salt, parmesan cheese, mozzarella cheese, coconut flour, dried basil, dried thyme, garlic powder, and stevia powder.

2. Get another mixing container and mix warm water, unsweetened almond milk, melted unsalted butter, and extra virgin olive oil.

3. As per the instructions on the manual of your machine, pour the ingredients in the bread pan.

4. Place the bread pan in the machine, and select the basic bread setting, together with the bread size and crust type, if available, then press start once you have closed the lid of the machine.

5. When the bread is ready, using oven mitts, remove the bread pan from the machine. Use a stainless spatula to extract the bread from the pan and turn the pan upside down on a metallic rack where the bread will cool off before slicing it.

**Nutrition:** Calories 49, Fat 2 g, Carb 2 g, Protein 4 g

# 46. BLUE CHEESE ONION BREAD

## INGREDIENTS

- ½ cup of blue cheese, crumbled
- 1 tsp. unsalted melted butter
- 1 tsp. fresh rosemary, chopped
- 1 ½ cup of almond fine flour
- 3 teaspoons olive oil extra virgin
- 1 teaspoon baking powder
- ½ cup warm water
- 1 yellow onion sliced and sautéed in butter until golden brown
- 2 garlic cloves, crushed
- 1 teaspoon Swerve sweetener
- 1 teaspoon salt

 **PREPARATION** 5 MIN    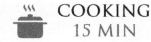 **COOKING** 15 MIN    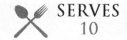 **SERVES** 10

## DIRECTIONS

1. Prepare a mixing container, where you will combine the almond flour, swerve sweetener, baking powder, freshly chopped rosemary, crumbled blue cheese, sautéed sliced onion, salt, and crushed garlic.
2. Get another container, where you will combine the warm water, melted butter, and extra virgin olive oil.
3. As per the instructions on the manual of your machine, pour the ingredients in the bread pan.
4. Place the bread pan in the machine, and select the basic bread setting, together with the bread size and crust type, if available, then press start once you have closed the lid of the machine.
5. When the bread is ready, using oven mitts, remove the bread pan from the machine.
6. Use a stainless spatula to extract the bread from the pan, and turn the pan upside down on a metallic rack where the bread will cool off before slicing it.
7.

**Nutrition:** Calories 100, Fat 6 g, Carb 3 g, Protein 11 g

# 47. LOW-CARB BAGEL

## INGREDIENTS

**For Bagel:**
- 1 cup Protein powder, unflavored
- 1/3 cup coconut flour
- 1 tsp. Baking powder
- ½ tsp. Sea salt
- ¼ cup ground flaxseed
- 1/3 cup sour cream
- 12 eggs

**Seasoning topping:**
- 1 tsp. Dried parsley
- 1 tsp. Dried oregano
- 1 tsp. Dried minced onion
- ½ tsp. Garlic powder
- ½ tsp. Dried basil
- ½ tsp. Sea salt

 **PREPARATION** 15 MIN      **COOKING** 25 MIN     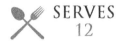 **SERVES** 12

## DIRECTIONS

1. In a mixer, blend sour cream and eggs until well combined.
2. Whisk together the flaxseed, salt, baking powder, Protein powder, and coconut flour in a bowl.
3. Whisk the topping seasoning together in a small bowl. Set aside.
4. Following the instructions on your machine's manual, mix the dry ingredients into the wet ingredients and pour in the bread pan, taking care to follow how to mix in the baking powder.
5. Place the bread pan in the machine, and select the basic bread setting, together with the bread size and crust type, if available, then press start once you have closed the lid of the machine.
6. When the bread is ready, using oven mitts, remove the bread pan from the machine.
7. Sprinkle pan with about 1 tsp. Topping seasoning and evenly pour batter into each.
8. Let the bread cool before slice it.
9. Sprinkle the top of each bagel evenly with the rest of the seasoning mixture.
10. Serve.

**Nutrition:** Calories 134, Fat 6.8 g, Carb 4.2 g, Protein 12.1 g

# 48. CHEDDAR SAUSAGE MUFFINS

## INGREDIENTS

- 6 oz. Cooked sausage, grease drained, thinly sliced
- ¼ cup water
- 1 tbsp. baking powder
- ¼ cup heavy cream
- 1 cup shredded sharp white cheddar cheese
- 1 ½ cups almond flour
- ½ tsp. Italian seasoning
- ½ tsp. Sea salt
- 1 tbsp. Chopped fresh chives
- 2 minced large garlic cloves
- 1 large egg
- 4 oz. Softened cream cheese

 **PREPARATION**
15 MIN

 **COOKING**
25 MIN

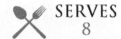 **SERVES**
8

## DIRECTIONS

1. Using a hand mixer on low speed, whip the eggs and cream cheese in a bowl.
2. Add the garlic, chives, sea salt, Italian seasoning, then mix into the egg cheese mixture.
3. Add the water, almond flour, heavy cream, and cheddar cheese. Mix well.
4. Slowly mix in the sausage into the mixture using a spatula.
5. However, take a look to the manufacturer's instructions for mixing dry and wet ingredients.
6. Pour mixture in the bread machine loaf pan.
7. Place the bread pan in the machine, and select the dough cycle setting, or specific muffin program, if available.
8. Then press start once you have closed the lid of the machine.
9. Remove dough from bread machine when cycle is complete.
10. Preheat the oven to 350 F
11. Lightly grease muffin pan with cooking spray.
12. Drop a heap mold of dough into 8 wells on the muffin top pan.
13. Bake in the oven for 25 minutes.
14. Cool and serve.

**Nutrition:** Calories 321, Fat 28 g, Carb 3.5 g, Protein 13 g

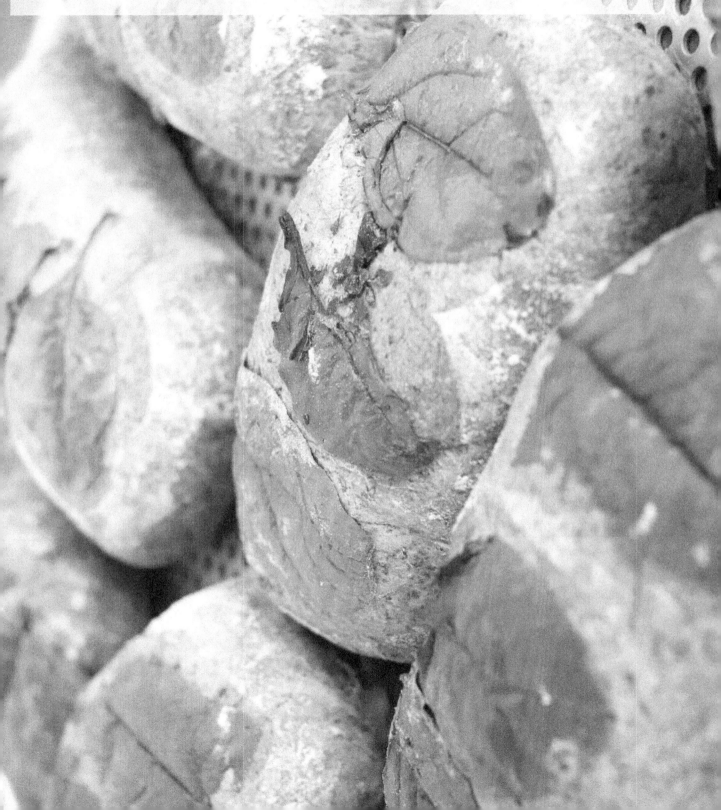

# CHAPTER 10: VEGETABLE BREAD RECIPES

# 49. HEARTY CHEESY BROCCOLI BREAD

## INGREDIENTS

- 5 eggs, whisked
- 2 teaspoons baking powder
- 1 cup cheddar, shredded
- 1 cup broccoli florets, separated
- 4 tablespoons coconut flour
- Cooking spray

 **PREPARATION** 10 MIN           **COOKING** 30 MIN          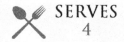 **SERVES** 4

## DIRECTIONS

1. In a bowl, mix all the ingredients except the cooking spray and stir the batter really well.
2. Pour batter in the bread machine pan pre-greased with cooking spray.
3. Set the bread machine to the basic bread setting.
4. When the bread is done, remove bread machine pan from the bread machine.
5. Let cool slightly before transferring to a cooling rack.
6. Cool the bread down, slice and serve.

**Nutrition:** Calories 123, Fat 6 g, Fiber 1 g, Carbs 3 g, Protein 6 g

# 50. KETO SPINACH BREAD

## INGREDIENTS

- ½ cup spinach, chopped
- 1 tablespoon olive oil
- 1 cup water
- 3 cups almond flour
- A pinch of salt and black pepper
- 1 tablespoon stevia
- 1 teaspoon baking powder
- 1 teaspoon baking soda
- ½ cup cheddar, shredded

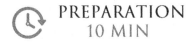 **PREPARATION** 10 MIN     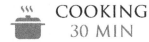 **COOKING** 30 MIN     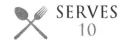 **SERVES** 10

## DIRECTIONS

1. Use a small mixing bowl to combine the flour, with salt, pepper, stevia, baking powder, baking soda and the cheddar and stir well.
2. In the bread machine pan add all wet Ingredients.
3. Add all of your dry Ingredients, from the small mixing bowl, in the bread machine pan.
4. Set the bread machine to the basic bread setting.
5. When the bread is done, remove bread machine pan from the bread machine.
6. Let cool slightly before transferring to a cooling rack.
7. Slice and serve.

**Nutrition:** Calories 142, Fat 7 g, Fiber 3 g, Carbs 5 g, Protein 6 g

# 51. CINNAMON ASPARAGUS BREAD

## INGREDIENTS

- 1 teaspoon stevia
- ¾ cup coconut oil, melted
- 1 and ½ cups almond flour
- 2 eggs, whisked
- A pinch of salt
- 1 teaspoon baking soda
- 1 teaspoon cinnamon powder
- 2 cups asparagus, chopped
- Cooking spray

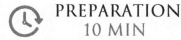 **PREPARATION** 10 MIN

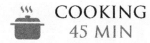 **COOKING** 45 MIN

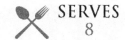 **SERVES** 8

## DIRECTIONS

1. In a bowl, mix all the ingredients except the cooking spray and stir the batter really well.
2. Pour batter in the bread machine pan pre-greased with cooking spray.
3. Set the bread machine to the basic bread setting.
4. When the bread is done, remove bread machine pan from the bread machine.
5. Let cool slightly before transferring to a cooling rack.
6. Cool the bread down, slice and serve.

**Nutrition:** Calories 165, Fat 6 g, Fiber 3 g, Carbs 5 g, Protein 7 g

# 52. KALE AND CHEESE BREAD

## INGREDIENTS

- 2 cups kale, chopped
- 1 cup warm water
- 1 teaspoon baking powder
- 1 teaspoon baking soda
- 2 tablespoons olive oil
- 2 teaspoons stevia
- 1 cup parmesan, grated
- 3 cups almond flour
- A pinch of salt
- 1 egg
- 2 tablespoons basil, chopped

 **PREPARATION**
10 MIN

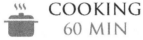 **COOKING**
60 MIN

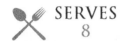 **SERVES**
8

## DIRECTIONS

1. In a bowl, mix the flour, salt, parmesan, stevia, baking soda and baking powder and stir.
2. Pour batter in the bread machine pan pre-greased with cooking spray.
3. Add the rest of the ingredients gradually and following order in manufacturer's manual instructions
4. Set the bread machine to the basic bread setting.
5. When the bread is done, remove bread machine pan from the bread machine.
6. Let cool slightly before transferring to a cooling rack.
7. Cool the bread down, slice and serve.

**Nutrition:** Calories 231, Fat 7 g, Fiber 2 g, Carbs 5 g, Protein 7 g

# 53. BEET BREAD

## INGREDIENTS

- 1 cup warm water
- 3 ½ cups almond flour
- 1 and ½ cups beet puree
- 2 tablespoons olive oil
- A pinch of salt
- 1 teaspoon stevia
- 1 teaspoon baking powder
- 1 teaspoon baking soda

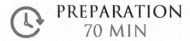 **PREPARATION**
70 MIN

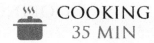 **COOKING**
35 MIN

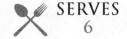 **SERVES**
6

## DIRECTIONS

1. Add all ingredients gradually in the bread machine's pan, following the manufacturer's instructions for mixing dry and wet ingredients.
2. Set the bread machine to the basic bread setting.
3. When the bread is done, remove bread machine pan from the bread machine.
4. Let cool slightly before transferring to a cooling rack.
5. Cool the bread down, slice and serve.

**Nutrition:** Calories 200, Fat 8 g, Fiber 3 g, Carbs 5 g, Protein 6 g

# 54. KETO CELERY BREAD

## INGREDIENTS

- ½ cup celery, chopped
- 3 cups almond flour
- 1 teaspoon baking powder
- 1 teaspoon baking soda
- A pinch of salt
- 2 tablespoons coconut oil, melted
- ½ cup celery puree

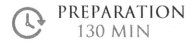 **PREPARATION**
130 MIN

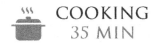 **COOKING**
35 MIN

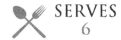 **SERVES**
6

## DIRECTIONS

1. Add all ingredients gradually in the bread machine's pan, following the manufacturer's instructions for mixing dry and wet ingredients.
2. Set the bread machine to the basic bread setting.
3. When the bread is done, remove bread machine pan from the bread machine.
4. Let cool slightly before transferring to a cooling rack.
5. Cool the bread down, slice and serve.

**Nutrition:** Calories 162, Fat 6 g, Fiber 2 g, Carbs 6 g, Protein 4 g

# 55. EASY CUCUMBER BREAD

## INGREDIENTS

- 1 cup erythritol
- 1 cup coconut oil, melted
- 1 cup almonds, chopped
- 1 teaspoon vanilla extract
- A pinch of salt
- A pinch of nutmeg, ground
- ½ teaspoon baking powder
- A pinch of cloves
- 3 eggs
- 1 teaspoon baking soda
- 1 tablespoon cinnamon powder
- 2 cups cucumber, peeled, deseeded and shredded
- 3 cups coconut flour
- Cooking spray

 **PREPARATION** 10 MIN     **COOKING** 50 MIN    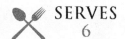 **SERVES** 6

## DIRECTIONS

1. In a bowl, mix the flour with cucumber, cinnamon, baking soda, cloves, baking powder, nutmeg, salt, vanilla extract and the almonds and stir well.
2. Add the rest of the ingredients, stir well and transfer the dough in the bread machine loaf pan pre-greased with cooking spray.
3. However, take a look to the manufacturer's instructions for mixing dry and wet ingredients.
4. Place the bread pan in the machine, and select the basic bread setting, together with the bread size, if available, then press start once you have closed the lid of the machine.
5. When the bread is ready, using oven mitts, remove the bread pan from the machine.
6. Cool and serve.

**Nutrition:** Calories 243, Fat 12 g, Fiber 3 g, Carbs 6 g, Protein 7 g

# 56. RED BELL PEPPER BREAD

## INGREDIENTS

- 1 ½ cups red bell peppers, chopped
- 1 teaspoon baking powder
- 1 teaspoon baking soda
- 2 tablespoons warm water
- 1 and ¼ cups parmesan, grated
- A pinch of salt
- 4 cups almond flour
- 2 tablespoons ghee, melted
- 1/3 cup almond milk
- 1 egg

 **PREPARATION** 10 MIN    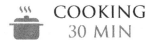 **COOKING** 30 MIN    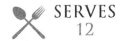 **SERVES** 12

## DIRECTIONS

1. In a bowl, mix the flour with salt, parmesan, baking powder, baking soda and the bell peppers and stir well.
2. Add the rest of the ingredients, stir well and transfer the dough in the bread machine loaf pan pre-greased with cooking spray.
3. However, take a look to the manufacturer's instructions for mixing dry and wet ingredients.
4. Place the bread pan in the machine, and select the basic bread setting, together with the bread size, if available, then press start once you have closed the lid of the machine.
5. When the bread is ready, using oven mitts, remove the bread pan from the machine.
6. Cool and serve.

**Nutrition:** Calories 100, Fat 5 g, Fiber 1 g, Carbs 4 g, Protein 4 g

# 57. TOMATO BREAD

## INGREDIENTS

- 6 cups almond flour
- ½ teaspoon basil, dried
- ¼ teaspoon rosemary, dried
- 1 teaspoon oregano, dried
- ½ teaspoon garlic powder
- 2 tablespoons olive oil
- 2 cups tomato juice
- ½ cup tomato sauce
- 1 teaspoon baking powder
- 1 teaspoon baking soda
- 3 tablespoons swerve

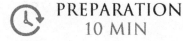 **PREPARATION** 10 MIN

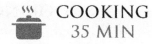 **COOKING** 35 MIN

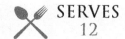 **SERVES** 12

## DIRECTIONS

1. In a bowl, mix the flour with basil, rosemary, oregano and garlic and stir.
2. Add the rest of the ingredients, stir well and transfer the dough in the bread machine loaf pan pre-greased with cooking spray.
3. However, take a look to the manufacturer's instructions for mixing dry and wet ingredients.
4. Place the bread pan in the machine, and select the basic bread setting, together with the bread size, if available, then press start once you have closed the lid of the machine.
5. When the bread is ready, using oven mitts, remove the bread pan from the machine.
6. Cool down and serve.

**Nutrition:** Calories 102, Fat 5 g, Fiber 3 g, Carbs 7 g, Protein 4 g

# 58. HERBED GARLIC BREAD

## INGREDIENTS

- ½ cup coconut flour
- 8 tbsp. melted butter, cooled
- tsp. baking powder
- 6 large eggs
- 1 tsp. garlic powder
- tsp. rosemary, dried
- ¼ tsp. salt
- ½ tsp. onion powder

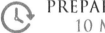 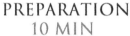 **PREPARATION**
**10 MIN**

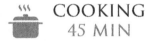 **COOKING**
**45 MIN**

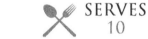 **SERVES**
**10**

## DIRECTIONS

1. Prepare bread machine loaf pan greasing it with cooking spray.
2. In a bowl, add coconut flour, baking powder, onion, garlic, rosemary, and salt into a bowl. Combine and mix well.
3. Into another bowl, add eggs and beat until bubbly on top.
4. Add melted butter into the bowl with the eggs and beat until mixed.
5. Following the instructions on your machine's manual, mix the dry ingredients into the wet ingredients and pour in the bread machine loaf pan, taking care to follow how to mix in the baking powder.
6. Place the bread pan in the machine, and select the basic bread setting, together with the bread size and crust type, if available, then press start once you have closed the lid of the machine.
7. When the bread is ready, using oven mitts, remove the bread pan from the machine.
8. Let it cool before slicing.
9. Cool, slice, and enjoy.

**Nutrition Facts per Serving:** Calories 147, Fat 12.5 g, Carb 3.5 g, Protein 4.6 g

# 59. HERBED KETO BREAD

## INGREDIENTS

- 3 cups coconut flour
- 1 teaspoon baking powder
- 1 teaspoon baking soda
- 2 teaspoons stevia
- 1 ½ cups warm water
- ½ teaspoon basil, dried
- 1 teaspoon oregano, dried
- ½ teaspoon thyme, dried
- ½ teaspoon marjoram, dried
- 2 tablespoons olive oil

 **PREPARATION**
90 MIN

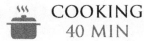 **COOKING**
40 MIN

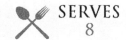 **SERVES**
8

## DIRECTIONS

1. In a bowl, mix the flour with baking powder, baking soda, stevia, basil, oregano, thyme, and the marjoram and stir.
2. Add the rest of the ingredients, stir well and transfer the dough in the bread machine loaf pan pre-greased with cooking spray.
3. However, take a look to the manufacturer's instructions for mixing dry and wet ingredients.
4. Place the bread pan in the machine, and select the basic bread setting, together with the bread size, if available, then press start once you have closed the lid of the machine.
5. When the bread is ready, using oven mitts, remove the bread pan from the machine.
6. Cool the bread down before serving.

**Nutrition:** Calories 200, Fat 7 g, Fiber 3 g, Carbs 5 g, Protein 6 g

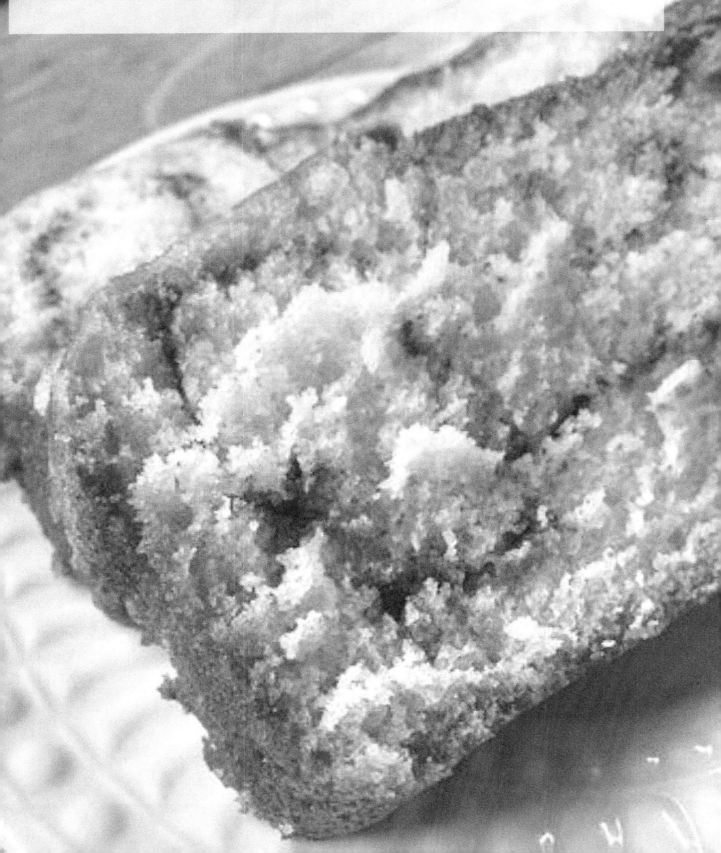

# 60. CINNAMON BREAD

## INGREDIENTS

- 3 tablespoons sour cream
- 3 eggs, pasteurized
- 2 teaspoons vanilla extract, unsweetened
- ¼ cup / 60 grams melted butter, grass-fed, unsalted
- 2 cups / 200 grams almond flour
- 1/3 cup / 65 grams erythritol sweetener
- 2 tablespoons cinnamon
- 1 teaspoon baking soda
- 1 teaspoon baking powder

 **PREPARATION**
10 MIN

 **COOKING**
4 HOURS

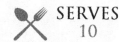 **SERVES**
10

## DIRECTIONS

1. Gather all the ingredients for the bread and plug in the bread machine having the capacity of 2 pounds of bread recipe.

2. Take a large bowl, place sour cream in it and then beat in eggs, vanilla, and butter until combined.

3. Take a separate large bowl, place flour in it, and then stir in sweetener, cinnamon, baking powder, and soda until mixed.

4. Add egg mixture into the bread bucket, top with flour mixture, shut the lid, select the "basic/white" cycle setting and then press the up/down arrow button to adjust baking time according to your bread machine; it will take 3 to 4 hours.

5. Then press the crust button to select light crust if available, and press the "start/stop" button to switch on the bread machine.

6. When the bread machine beeps, open the lid, then take out the bread basket and lift out the bread.

7. Let bread cool on a wire rack for 1 hour, then cut it into ten slices and serve.

**Nutrition:** Cal 169, Fat 14.5 g, Protein 5.4 g, Carb 5.2, Fiber 2 g, Net Carb 2.2 g

# 61. BANANA BREAD

## INGREDIENTS

- 2 eggs, pasteurized
- 1 teaspoon banana extract, unsweetened
- ¼ cup / 50 grams erythritol sweetener
- 3 tablespoons butter, grass-fed, unsalted, softened
- 2 tablespoons almond milk, unsweetened
- 1 cup / 100 grams almond flour
- 2 tablespoons coconut flour

- ¼ cup / 50 grams walnuts, chopped
- 1 teaspoons baking powder
- ¼ teaspoon xanthan gum
- ⅛ teaspoon of sea salt
- 1 teaspoon cinnamon

 **PREPARATION**
10 MIN

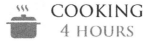 **COOKING**
4 HOURS

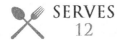 **SERVES**
12

## DIRECTIONS

1. Gather all the ingredients for the bread and plug in the bread machine having the capacity of 2 pounds of bread recipe.
2. Take a large bowl, crack eggs in it and then beat in the banana extract, sweetener, butter, and milk until blended.
3. Take a separate large bowl, place flours in it, and then stir in remaining ingredients until mixed.
4. Add egg mixture into the bread bucket, top with flour mixture, shut the lid, select the "basic/white" cycle setting and then press the up/down arrow button to adjust baking time according to your bread machine; it will take 3 to 4 hours.
5. Then press the crust button to select light crust if available, and press the "start/stop" button to switch on the bread machine.
6. When the bread machine beeps, open the lid, then take out the bread basket and lift out the bread.
7. Let bread cool on a wire rack for 1 hour, then cut it into twelve slices and serve.

**Nutrition:** 240 Cal, 21 g Fat, 8.5 g Protein, 6.8 g Carb, 4.2 g Fiber, 2.6 g Net Carb

# 62. LEMON RASPBERRY LOAF

## INGREDIENTS

- 2 eggs, pasteurized
- 4 tablespoons sour cream
- 1 teaspoon vanilla extract, unsweetened
- 1 teaspoon lemon extract, unsweetened
- 4 tablespoons butter, grass-fed, unsalted, melted
- ¼ cup / 50 grams erythritol sweetener
- 2 tablespoons lemon juice
- ½ cup / 100 grams raspberries preserves
- 2 cups / 200 grams almond flour
- 1 ½ teaspoons baking powder

 **PREPARATION** 10 MIN

 **COOKING** 4 HOURS

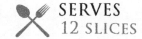 **SERVES** 12 SLICES

## DIRECTIONS

1. Gather all the ingredients for the bread and plug in the bread machine having the capacity of 2 pounds of bread recipe.
2. Take a large bowl, place flour in it, and then stir in baking soda until mixed.
3. Take a separate large bowl, crack eggs in it, beat in sour cream, extracts, butter, sweetener, and lemon juice until blended and then stir in raspberry preserve until just combined.
4. Add egg mixture into the bread bucket, top with flour mixture, shut the lid, select the "basic/white" cycle setting and then press the up/down arrow button to adjust baking time according to your bread machine; it will take 3 to 4 hours.
5. Then press the crust button to select light crust if available, and press the "start/stop" button to switch on the bread machine.
6. When the bread machine beeps, open the lid, then take out the bread basket and lift out the bread.
7. Let bread cool on a wire rack for 1 hour, then cut it and serve.

**Nutrition:** Cal 171, Fat 14,3 g, Protein 4.6 g, Carb 5 g, Fiber 2.4 g, Net Carb 2.6 g

# 63. WALNUT BREAD

## INGREDIENTS

- 4 eggs, pasteurized
- 2 tablespoons apple cider vinegar
- 4 tablespoons coconut oil
- ½ cup / 120 ml lukewarm water
- 1 cup / 200 grams walnuts chopped
- ½ cup / 65 grams coconut flour
- 1 tablespoon baking powder
- 2 tablespoons psyllium husk powder
- ½ teaspoon salt

 **PREPARATION** 10 MIN     **COOKING** 4 HOURS    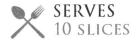 **SERVES** 10 SLICES

## DIRECTIONS

1. Gather all the ingredients for the bread and plug in the bread machine having the capacity of 2 pounds of bread recipe.
2. Take a large bowl, crack eggs in it, beat in vinegar, oil, and water until blended and stir in walnuts until just mixed.
3. Take a separate large bowl, place flour in it, and then stir in baking powder, husk powder, and salt until mixed.
4. Add egg mixture into the bread bucket, top with flour mixture, shut the lid, select the "basic/white" cycle setting and then press the up/down arrow button to adjust baking time according to your bread machine; it will take 3 to 4 hours.
5. Then press the crust button to select light crust if available, and press the "start/stop" button to switch on the bread machine.
6. When the bread machine beeps, open the lid, then take out the bread basket and lift out the bread.
7. Let bread cool on a wire rack for 1 hour, then cut it into ten slices and serve.

**Nutrition:** Cal 201, Fat 8.1 g, Protein 6 g, Carb 7.5 g, Fiber 4.7 g, Net Carb 2.8

# 64. ALMOND BUTTER BREAD

## INGREDIENTS

- 3 eggs, pasteurized
- 1 cup / 225 grams almond butter
- 1 tablespoon apple cider vinegar
- ½ teaspoon baking soda

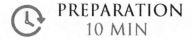 **PREPARATION** 10 MIN
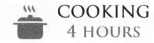 **COOKING** 4 HOURS
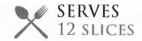 **SERVES** 12 SLICES

## DIRECTIONS

1. Gather all the ingredients for the bread and plug in the bread machine having the capacity of 1 pound of bread recipe.
2. Crack eggs in a bowl and then beat in butter, vinegar, and baking soda until combined.
3. Add egg mixture into the bread bucket, shut the lid, select the "basic/white" cycle setting and then press the up/down arrow button to adjust baking time according to your bread machine; it will take 3 to 4 hours.
4. Then press the crust button to select light crust if available, and press the "start/stop" button to switch on the bread machine.
5. When the bread machine beeps, open the lid, then take out the bread basket and lift out the bread.
6. Let bread cool on a wire rack for 1 hour, then cut it into twelve slices and serve.

**Nutrition:** Cal 152, Fat 13 g, Protein 6.4 g, Carb 5.6 g, Fiber 3.1 g, Net Carb 2.1 g

# 65. CHOCOLATE ZUCCHINI BREAD

## INGREDIENTS

- 1 cup / 200 grams grated zucchini, moisture squeezed thoroughly
- 1/3 cup / 60 grams ground flaxseed
- ½ cup / 100 grams almond flour
- ½ teaspoon salt
- 2 ½ teaspoons baking powder
- 1 ¼ tablespoon psyllium husk powder
- 1/3 cup / 60 grams of cocoa powder
- 4 eggs, pasteurized
- 1 tablespoon coconut cream
- 5 tablespoons coconut oil
- ¾ cup / 150 grams erythritol sweetener
- 1 teaspoon vanilla extract, unsweetened
- ½ cup / 115 grams sour cream
- ½ cup / 100 grams chocolate chips, unsweetened

 **PREPARATION** 10 MIN      **COOKING** 4 HOURS     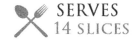 **SERVES** 14 SLICES

## DIRECTIONS

1. Wrap zucchini in cheesecloth and twist well until all the moisture is released, set aside until required.
2. Gather all the ingredients for the bread and plug in the bread machine having the capacity of 2 pounds of bread recipe.
3. Take a large bowl, place flaxseed and flour in it, and then stir salt, baking powder, husk, and cocoa powder in it until mixed.
4. Take a separate large bowl, crack eggs in it and then beat in coconut cream, coconut oil, sweetener, and vanilla until combined.
5. Blend in half of the flour mixture, then sour cream and remaining half of flour mixture until incorporated and then fold in chocolate chips until mixed.
6. Add batter into the bread bucket, shut the lid, select the "basic/white" cycle setting and then press the up/down arrow button to adjust baking time according to your bread machine; it will take 3 to 4 hours.
7. Then press the crust button to select light crust if available, and press the "start/stop" button to switch on the bread machine.

8. When the bread machine beeps, open the lid, then take out the bread basket and lift out the bread.

9. Let bread cool on a wire rack for 1 hour, then cut it into fourteen slices and serve.

**Nutrition:** Cal 187, Fat 15.9 g, Protein 6.2 g, Carb 8.8 g, Fiber 5.2 g, Net Carb 3.6 g

# 66. PUMPKIN BREAD

## INGREDIENTS

- 2 eggs, pasteurized
- 1 cup / 225 grams almond butter, unsweetened
- 2/3 cup / 130 grams erythritol sweetener
- 2/3 cup / 150 grams pumpkin puree
- 1/8 teaspoon ground cloves
- 1/2 teaspoon ground cinnamon
- 1/8 teaspoon ground ginger

- 1 teaspoon baking powder
- 1/2 teaspoon ground nutmeg

 **PREPARATION**
10 MIN

 **COOKING**
4 HOURS

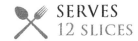 **SERVES**
12 SLICES

## DIRECTIONS

1. Gather all the ingredients for the bread and plug in the bread machine having the capacity of 2 pounds of bread recipe.

2. Take a large bowl, crack eggs in it and then beat in remaining ingredients in it in the order described in the ingredients until incorporated.

3. Add batter into the bread bucket, shut the lid, select the "basic/white" cycle setting and then press the up/down arrow

button to adjust baking time according to your bread machine; it will take 3 to 4 hours.

4. Then press the crust button to select light crust if available, and press the "start/stop" button to switch on the bread machine.

5. When the bread machine beeps, open the lid, then take out the bread basket and lift out the bread.

6. Let bread cool on a wire rack for 1 hour, then cut it into twelve slices and serve.

**Nutrition:** Cal 150, Fat 12.9 g, Protein 6.7 g, Carb 7 g, Fiber 2 g, Net Carb 5 g

# 67. STRAWBERRY BREAD

## INGREDIENTS

- 5 eggs, pasteurized
- 1 egg white, pasteurized
- 1 ½ teaspoons vanilla extract, unsweetened
- 2 tablespoons heavy whipping cream
- 2 tablespoons sour cream
- 1 cup monk fruit powder
- 1 ½ teaspoons baking powder
- ½ teaspoon salt

- ½ teaspoon cinnamon
- 8 tablespoons butter, melted
- ¾ cup / 100 grams coconut flour
- ¾ cup / 150 grams chopped strawberries

 **PREPARATION** 10 MIN      **COOKING** 4 HOURS     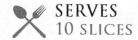 **SERVES** 10 SLICES

## DIRECTIONS

1. Gather all the ingredients for the bread and plug in the bread machine having the capacity of 2 pounds of bread recipe.
2. Take a large bowl, crack eggs in it and then beat in egg white, vanilla, heavy cream, sour cream, baking powder, salt, and cinnamon until well combined.
3. Then stir in coconut flour and fold in strawberries until mixed.
4. Add batter into the bread bucket, shut the lid, select the "basic/white" cycle or "low-carb" setting and then press the

up/down arrow button to adjust baking time according to your bread machine; it will take 3 to 4 hours.
5. Then press the crust button to select light crust if available, and press the "start/stop" button to switch on the bread machine.
6. When the bread machine beeps, open the lid, then take out the bread basket and lift out the bread.
7. Let bread cool on a wire rack for 1 hour, then cut it into ten slices and serve.

**Nutrition:** Cal 201, Fat 16.4 g, Protein 4.7 g, Carb 6.1 g, Fiber 3 g, Net Carb 3.1 g

# 68. BLUEBERRY BREAD LOAF

## INGREDIENTS

**For the bread dough:**
- 10 tbsp. coconut flour
- 9 tbsp. melted butter
- 2/3 cup granulates swerve sweetener
- ½ tsp. baking powder
- 1 tbsp. heavy whipping cream
- 1 ½ tsp. vanilla extract
- ½ tsp. cinnamon
- 3 tbsp. sour cream

- 6 large eggs
- ½ tsp. salt
- ¾ cup blueberries

**For the topping:**
- 2 tbsp. heavy whipping cream
- 1 tbsp. swerve sweetener
- 1 tsp. melted butter
- 1/8 tsp. vanilla extract
- ¼ tsp. lemon zest

 **PREPARATION** 20 MIN

 **COOKING** 65 MIN

 **SERVES** 12

## DIRECTIONS

1. Gather all the ingredients for the bread and plug in the bread machine having the capacity of 2 pounds of bread recipe.
2. Take a large bowl, crack eggs in it and then beat in cream, butter, and vanilla until combined.
3. Take a separate large bowl, place coconut flour in it, then stir in sweetener and baking powder until mixed and fold in blueberries.
4. Add egg mixture into the bread bucket, top with flour mixture, shut the lid, select the "basic/white" cycle or "low-carb" setting and then press the up/down arrow button to adjust baking time according to your bread machine; it will take 3 to 4 hours.
5. Then press the crust button to select light crust if available, and press the "start/stop" button to switch on the bread machine.
6. When the bread machine beeps, open the lid, then take out the bread basket and lift out the bread.
7. Meanwhile, in a bowl, beat the vanilla extract, butter, heavy whipping cream, lemon zest, and confectioner swerve. Mix until creamy.

**8.** Then drizzle the icing topping on the bread.

**9.** Enjoy.

**Nutrition:** Calories 155, Fat 13 g, Carb 4 g, Protein 3 g

# 69. CRANBERRY AND ORANGE BREAD

## INGREDIENTS

- 1 cup / 200 grams chopped cranberries
- 2/3 cup and 3 tablespoons / 175 grams monk fruit powder, divided
- 5 eggs, pasteurized
- 1 egg white, pasteurized
- 2 tablespoons sour cream
- 1 ½ teaspoons orange extract, unsweetened
- 1 teaspoon vanilla extract, unsweetened
- 9 tablespoons butter, grass-fed, unsalted, melted
- 9 tablespoons coconut flour
- 1 ½ teaspoons baking powder
- ¼ teaspoon salt

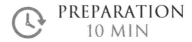 **PREPARATION** 10 MIN

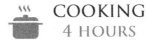 **COOKING** 4 HOURS

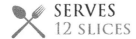 **SERVES** 12 SLICES

## DIRECTIONS

1. Take a small bowl, place cranberries in it, and then stir in 4 tablespoons of monk fruit powder until combined, set aside until required.

2. Gather all the ingredients for the bread and plug in the bread machine having the capacity of 2 pounds of bread recipe.

3. Take a large bowl, crack eggs in it, beat in remaining ingredients in it in the order described in the ingredients until incorporated and then fold in cranberries until just mixed.

4. Add batter into the bread bucket, shut the lid, select the "basic/white" cycle or "low-carb" setting and then press the up/down arrow button to adjust baking time according to your bread machine; it will take 3 to 4 hours.

5. Then press the crust button to select light crust if available, and press the "start/stop" button to switch on the bread machine.

6. When the bread machine beeps, open the lid, then take out the bread basket and lift out the bread.

7. Let bread cool on a wire rack for 1 hour, then cut it into twelve slices and serve

**Nutrition:** Cal 149, Fat 13.1 g, Protein 3.9 g, Carb 4 g, Fiber 1.5 g, Net Carb 2.5 g

# 70. BLUEBERRY BREAD

## INGREDIENTS

- 4 eggs, pasteurized
- 3 tablespoons heavy whipping cream
- 3 tablespoons butter, grass-fed, unsalted, melted
- 1 teaspoon vanilla extract, unsweetened
- 2 tablespoons coconut flour
- 2 cups / 200 grams almond flour
- ½ cup / 100 grams erythritol
- 1 ½ teaspoons baking powder
- 1 cup / 200 grams blueberries

 **PREPARATION**
10 MIN

 **COOKING**
4 HOURS

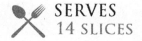 **SERVES**
14 SLICES

## DIRECTIONS

1. Gather all the ingredients for the bread and plug in the bread machine having the capacity of 2 pounds of bread recipe.
2. Take a large bowl, crack eggs in it and then beat in cream, butter, and vanilla until combined.
3. Take a separate large bowl, place flours in it, then stir in sweetener and baking powder until mixed and fold in blueberries.
4. Add egg mixture into the bread bucket, top with flour mixture, shut the lid, select the "basic/white" cycle or "low-carb" setting and then press the up/down arrow button to adjust baking time according to your bread machine; it will take 3 to 4 hours.
5. Then press the crust button to select light crust if available, and press the "start/stop" button to switch on the bread machine.
6. When the bread machine beeps, open the lid, then take out the bread basket and lift out the bread.
7. Let bread cool on a wire rack for 1 hour, then cut it into eleven slices and serve.

**Nutrition:** Cal 211, Fat 18.2 g, Protein 7.7 g, Carb 8.9 g, Fiber 3.7 g, Net Carb 5.2 g

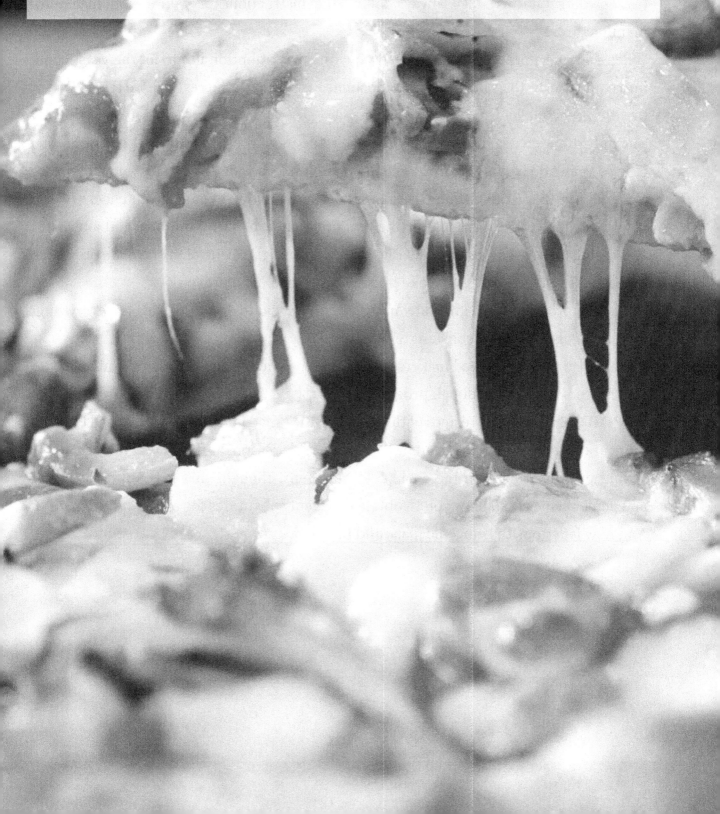

# CHAPTER 12: KETOGENIC PIZZA AND BREADSTICKS

In this chapter I will explain how to make pizza or breadsticks with the bread machine. It's a very convenient and easy method, because as usual, you just need to put the ingredients in the basket following the right sequence, putting first the liquids and then the powders (at this stage always follow the instructions of your bread machine's manufacturer).

When you make pizza with your bread machine, pay attention not to let the yeast come into contact with the salt (it could compromise leavening), the rest will be taken care of by your bread maker.

The only difference is the cooking you have to do in your kitchen oven., because in this case you can't do it with the bread machine... unless you want to get a tasty loaf of bread.

Generally, every bread machine has a program for pizza dough, make your checks before you start baking. It's a very interesting function that lasts 45-60 minutes and alternates processing phases with pause phases to allow leavening. It's one of my favorite programs because it's really amazing to make pizza to bake then in your oven.

Using this program has a great advantage, it allows you to dough and leaven everything in a single place and at a constant temperature.

For breadsticks many bread makers have also a specific setting. If it is not available, you can use cookies or pasta dough program.

**IMPORTANT**: in some recipes of this chapter, the bread maker will not be used because there are no ingredients to knead or leaven. For this reason, at first, I was undecided if I should put this section in the cookbook, but then I thought that it is still about tasty ketogenic recipes that allow you to obtain excellent substitutes for pizza. Try them!

And now let's go with ketogenic pizza and breadstick recipes!

# 71. DOUGH FOR YEAST KETO PIZZA (WITH GLUTEN)

## INGREDIENTS

- 1 ¼ cup super fine almond flour
- 1 cup plus 2 tablespoons warm (like bath water) water, divided
- 1 teaspoon sugar (needed to activate yeast)
- ½ teaspoon ground ginger
- ½ teaspoons active dry yeast
- 1 cup vital wheat gluten

- ½ teaspoon salt
- 1 ½ teaspoon baking powder
- 3 tablespoons extra virgin olive oil
- ½ tablespoon butter, melted

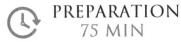 **PREPARATION** 75 MIN

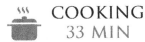 **COOKING** 33 MIN

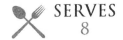 **SERVES** 8

## DIRECTIONS

1. Add all ingredients to bread machine pan following order in your bread machine's manual instructions, taking care on how to mix in the yeast.
2. Place the bread pan in the machine, and select the dough cycle setting, or specific pizza program, if available.
3. Then press start once you have closed the lid of the machine.
4. Remove dough from bread machine when cycle is complete.
5. Cover a large cookie sheet with parchment paper.

6. Form the dough into a ball and place it on the parchment covered cookie sheet. Press the dough and form it into a large circular crust (about 10 inches wide).
7. Pre-heat the oven for 2 minutes until the temperature reaches 100-110 degrees F.
8. Place the crust in the warm oven and allow to rise for 45 minutes.
9. Remove from the oven and pre-heat the oven to 375 degrees F.
10. Brush the crust with melted butter and bake for 12-15 minutes until crust is firm and just beginning to brown.

11. Remove the crust from the oven and turn the heat up to 450 degrees F.
12. Top your pizza with whatever you like and then pop it back into the 450 degree oven for another 6-8 minutes until the crust has browned and the cheese has melted.
13. Allow the pizza to cool on the pan for 10 minutes before cutting into 8 slices.

**IMPORTANT:** this recipe contains gluten, so be careful if you are intolerant or have celiac disease. Immediately after this, you will find the recipe for gluten-free version. However, if gluten doesn't bother you, the keto pizza you are going to obtain will be indistinguishable from the original version!

**Nutrition:** Calories 216, Fat 15 g, Carbohydrates 7 g, Fiber 3 g, Protein 16 g

# 72. GLUTEN-FREE KETO PIZZA YEAST DOUGH

## INGREDIENTS

- 1 ½ cups Almond Flour
- 1 ¼ tsp Xanthan Gum
- ¼ tsp Baking Powder
- 1 tsp Salt
- ½ tbsp Apple Cider Vinegar
- 1 tbsp Active Yeast
- ¼ cup Warm Water *for yeast
- 2 Egg Whites, room temperature
- 1 whole Egg, room temperature

 **PREPARATION** 30 MIN      **COOKING** 10 MIN     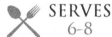 **SERVES** 6-8

## DIRECTIONS

1. Add all ingredients to bread machine pan fruit following order in your bread machine's manual instructions, taking care on how to mix in the yeast.

2. Place the bread pan in the machine, and select the dough cycle setting, or specific pizza program, if available.

3. Then press start once you have closed the lid of the machine.

4. Remove dough from bread machine when cycle is complete.

5. Place the dough onto a pizza pan lined with parchment and cover it with cling wrap, gently pressing into a flat round. You can roll up the edges for a high crust if you'd like.

6. Tent the dough with a clean cloth towel and allow to rise in a warm spot for 10-15 minutes.

7. Bake at 375° for 10-15 minutes or until the crust is golden.

8. If the sides are browning before the center, cover the edges with a bit of foil to prevent burning OR reduce the temperature to 325°/350° and bake an extra 5 minutes.

9. Add pizza toppings and return to a HOT oven (375) for 10-15 minutes.

**Nutrition:** Calories 180, Total Fat 15 g, Carbohydrates 7 g, Net Carbohydrates 4 g, Fiber 3 g, Protein 8 g

# 73. KETO UNLEAVENED PIZZA

## INGREDIENTS

- 2 eggs
- 2 tbsp. parmesan cheese
- 1 tbsp. psyllium husk powder
- ½ tsp. Italian seasoning
- salt
- 2 tsp. frying oil
- 1 ½ ounce mozzarella cheese
- 3 tbsp. tomato sauce
- 1 tbsp. chopped basil

 **PREPARATION** 10 MIN   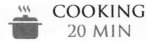 **COOKING** 20 MIN   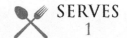 **SERVES** 1

## DIRECTIONS

**NOTE:** bread machine not required

1. In a blender, place the parmesan, psyllium husk powder, Italian seasoning, salt, and two eggs and blend.
2. Heat a large frying pan and add the oil.
3. Add the mixture to the pan in a large circular shape.
4. Flip once the underside is browning and then remove from the pan.
5. Spoon the tomato sauce onto the pizza crust and spread.
6. Add the cheese and spread over the top of the pizza.
7. Place the pizza into the oven – it is done once the cheese is melted.
8. Top the pizza with basil.

**Nutrition:** Calories 459, Fat 35 g, Carb 3.5 g, Protein 27 g

# 74. EASY ALMOND FLOUR PIZZA CRUST

## INGREDIENTS

- 2 cups almond flour
- 2 eggs
- 2 tbsp. coconut oil, melted
- ½ tsp. sea salt

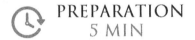 **PREPARATION**
5 MIN

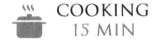 **COOKING**
15 MIN

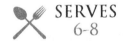 **SERVES**
6-8

## DIRECTIONS

1. Preheat the oven to 350F. Line a baking sheet with parchment paper.
2. Add all ingredients to bread machine pan fruit following order in your bread machine's manual instructions.
3. Place the bread pan in the machine, and select the dough cycle setting, or specific pizza program, if available.
4. Then press start once you have closed the lid of the machine.
5. Remove dough from bread machine when cycle is complete.
6. Form the dough into a ball. Put in between two parchment paper sheets, and roll out the dough to ¼ inch thick.
7. Remove the parchment paper piece on top. Place the crust on a pizza pan. Poke the crust with a toothpick a few times to prevent bubbling.
8. Bake for 15 to 20 minutes or until golden.
9. Top with your preferred toppings.
10. Return to the oven and bake for 10 to 15 minutes.
11. Serve.

**Nutrition:** Calories 211, Fat 19 g, Carb 3 g, Protein 8 g

# 75. PIZZA WITH A CHICKEN CRUST

## INGREDIENTS

- 7 ounces chicken breast meat, ground
- 7 ounces mozzarella cheese, grated
- 1 tsp. garlic salt
- 1 tsp. dried basil
- 4 tbsp. pizza topping sauce, no sugar added
- 4 ounces cheddar cheese, grated
- 12 slices pepperoni
- Fresh basil leaves

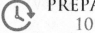 **PREPARATION** 10 MIN    **COOKING** 20 MIN   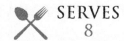 **SERVES** 8

## DIRECTIONS

**NOTE:** bread machine not required

1. Pre-heat the oven to 450F.
2. Line a 12-inch pizza pan with parchment.
3. Mix the chicken, cheese, garlic salt, and dried basil together.
4. Spread into the pizza pan in an even layer and bake in the preheated oven for 10 to 12 minutes.
5. Remove from the oven and cool a little before adding the topping of sauce, cheddar cheese, and pepperoni.
6. Once the topping is on, replace it in the hot oven and cook for 5 to 7 minutes or until hot and bubbly.
7. Remove from the oven and top with torn basil leaves.
8. Cut and serve.

**Nutrition:** Calories 228, Fat 14.6 g, Carb 3 g, Protein 20.2 g

# 76. KETO BREAKFAST PIZZA

## INGREDIENTS

- ½ tsp. salt
- 1 tbsp. psyllium husk powder
- 2 cups cauliflower florets, riced
- 2 tbsp. coconut flour
- 3 eggs

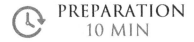 **PREPARATION** 10 MIN

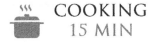 **COOKING** 15 MIN

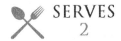 **SERVES** 2

## DIRECTIONS

**NOTE:** bread machine not required

1. Preheat the oven to 350F and line a baking tray with parchment paper.
2. In a bowl, add everything and mix well. Set aside for 5 minutes.
3. Then transfer into the baking tray. Flatten to give pizza dough shape.
4. Bake until golden brown, about 15 minutes.
5. Remove and top with toppings of your choice.
6. Serve.

**Nutrition:** Calories 454, Fat 31 g, Carb 8 g, Protein 22 g

# 77. THE BEST KETO PULL APART PIZZA BREAD RECIPE

## INGREDIENTS

- 2 ½ cups mozzarella cheese shredded
- 3 eggs beaten
- 1 ½ cup almond flour
- 1 tablespoon baking powder
- 2 oz. cream cheese
- ½ cup grated Parmesan cheese
- 1 teaspoon rosemary seasoning
- ½ cup shredded mild cheddar or a cheese or your choice
- ½ cup mini pepperoni slices
- 3-4 Sliced jalapeños
- Non-stick cooking spray

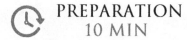 **PREPARATION** 10 MIN

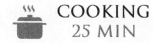 **COOKING** 25 MIN

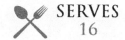 **SERVES** 16

## DIRECTIONS

1. Melt the Mozzarella cheese and cream cheese. You can do this on the stove top or for 1 minute in the microwave.
2. Add all ingredients to bread machine pan following order in your bread machine's manual instructions.
3. Place the bread pan in the machine, and select the dough cycle setting, or specific pizza program, if available.
4. Then press start once you have closed the lid of the machine.
5. Remove dough from bread machine when cycle is complete.
6. knead it until it forms into a sticky ball. I always use a silicone mat on the countertop to do this step.
7. Sprinkle the top of the dough with a small amount of parmesan cheese. This will help the dough not be so sticky when you start to handle it. I flip the dough over and sprinkle a small amount on the back side of the dough too.
8. Form the dough into a ball and cut it in half. Continue cutting the dough until you get about 16 pieces from each side, a total of 32 pieces total (give or take).

9. Roll the pieces of dough into equal sized balls then roll them in a plate of parmesan cheese that has been topped with a teaspoon of Rosemary seasoning. (This is the secret to forming the pull apart bread because the parmesan cheese coats each dough ball allowing it not to fully combine while it's baking. Plus, it adds an amazing flavor also.)
10. Spray the bundt pan with non-stick cooking spray.
11. Place the first layer of 16 prepared dough balls into a non-stick bundt pan.
12. Then add a layer of your favorite shredded cheese, mini pepperoni slices, and jalapeño if desired.
13. Add the next layer of 16 prepared dough balls on top of the first layer.
14. Top the last layer with the rest of the shredded cheese, mini pepperoni slices, and jalapeños.
15. Bake at 350°F for 25 minutes or until golden brown. It may take a bit longer if your bundt pan is thicker than the one I used.

**Nutrition:** Calories 142, Total Fat 9.4 g, Protein 11.1 g, Carbohydrates 3.5 g, Dietary Fiber 1.5 g, Sugar 0.8 g

# 78. MICROWAVE PEPPERONI PIZZA BREAD

## INGREDIENTS

- 1 tablespoon unsalted butter melted
- 1 large egg
- 1 tablespoon almond milk
- 1 tablespoon superfine almond flour
- 1 tablespoon coconut flour (not substitute with almond flour)

- 1/8 teaspoon baking powder
- 1/8 teaspoon Italian seasoning
- 1 tablespoon shredded parmesan cheese
- 1 tablespoon shredded mozzarella cheese
- 1 tablespoon low sugar tomato sauce optional
- 6-8 mini pepperoni

 **PREPARATION**
10 MIN

 **COOKING**
2 MIN

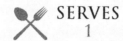 **SERVES**
1

## DIRECTIONS

**NOTE:** bread machine not required

1. In a large and wide (about 4 inches wide) microwave safe mug, add butter, egg, milk, almond flour, coconut flour, baking powder. Whisk until the batter is smooth.
2. Stir in Italian seasoning and Parmesan cheese.
3. Cook in the microwave at full power for about 90 seconds, or until the bread has cooked.
4. Spread tomato sauce (if using) over surface of bread.
5. Sprinkle mozzarella cheese over sauce.
6. Place mini pepperoni on top of the cheese.
7. Cook for an additional 30 seconds or until the cheese has melted.
8. Enjoy while still warm.

**Nutrition:** Nutrition: Calories 332, Total Fat 25.5 g, Saturated Fat 12.5 g, Protein 16.1 g, Carbohydrates 10.4 g, Dietary Fiber 4.3 g, Sugars 3.6 g

# 79. 5 MINUTES KETO PIZZA

## INGREDIENTS

**Pizza Crust:**
- 2 large eggs
- 2 tablespoons parmesan cheese
- 1 tablespoon psyllium husk powder
- ½ teaspoon Italian seasoning
- Salt to taste
- 2 teaspoons frying oil (you can use bacon fat)

**Topping:**
- 1 ½ oz. Mozzarella Cheese
- 3 tablespoons Rao's Tomato Sauce
- 1 tablespoon Freshly Chopped Basil

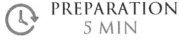 **PREPARATION** 5 MIN      **COOKING** 15 MIN     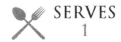 **SERVES** 1

## DIRECTIONS

**NOTE:** bread machine not required

1. In a bowl or container, use an immersion blender to mix together all the pizza crust ingredients.
2. Heat frying oil in a pan until hot, then spoon the mixture into the pan.
3. Spread out into a cirlce.
4. Once the edges have browned, flip and cook for 30-60 seconds on the other side.
5. Turn the stove off, and turn the broiler on.
6. Add tomato sauce and cheese, then broil for 1-2 minutes or until cheese is bubbling.

**Nutrition:** Calories 459, Total Fat 35 g, Protein 27 g, Carbohydrates 3.5 g, Dietary Fiber 9 g

# 80. ITSY BITSY PIZZA CRUSTS

## INGREDIENTS

**For dough:**
- 5 whole eggs and 3 egg whites
- ½ tsp. baking powder
- ¼ cup coconut flour sifted, with more for dusting
- Salt, pepper, Italian spices

**For sauce:**
- 2 garlic cloves, minced
- ½ cup organic tomato sauce
- 1 tsp. dried basil
- ¼ tsp. pink sea salt

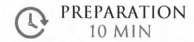 **PREPARATION**
10 MIN

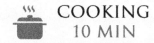 **COOKING**
10 MIN

 **SERVES**
2

## DIRECTIONS

1. Preheat oven to 350°F.
2. Add all dough ingredients to bread machine pan fruit following order in your bread machine's manual instructions.
3. Place the bread pan in the machine, and select the dough cycle setting, or specific pizza program, if available.
4. Then press start once you have closed the lid of the machine.
5. Remove dough from bread machine when cycle is complete.
6. Lightly grease a small pan and place over medium-low heat. Pour some of the batter evenly once the pan is hot.
7. 
8. Cover and let cook in oven for about 3-5minutes or until bubbles form on top. Flip the other side and cook for 2 minutes.
9. Transfer to a platter and repeat this for the remaining batter.
10. Once the crusts are cool, use a fork to roughly poke holes on the crusts. This will help them cook evenly.
11. Lightly dust with coconut flour and set aside.

**12.** For the sauce, whisk all the ingredients together then let stand for 30 minutes to allow thickening.

**13.** Spread the pizza bases with the sauce and top with your favorite toppings and bake for about 3-5 minutes or until done to desire.

**Nutrition:** Calories 125, Total Fat 1 g, Carb 6, Dietary Fiber 3 g, Protein 8 g, Cholesterol 34 mg, Sodium 89 mg

# 81. SIMPLE KETO PIZZA CRUST

## INGREDIENTS

- 100 g blanched almond flour
- 3 tablespoons coconut flour
- 2 tapioca flour
- 2 teaspoons baking powder
- ¼ teaspoon pink sea salt
- 2 teaspoons apple cider vinegar
- ¼ cup water
- 1 egg

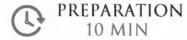 **PREPARATION** 10 MIN

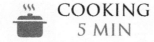 **COOKING** 5 MIN

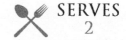 **SERVES** 2

## DIRECTIONS

1. Add all ingredients to bread machine pan fruit following order in your bread machine's manual instructions.
2. Place the bread pan in the machine, and select the dough cycle setting, or specific pizza program, if available.
3. Then press start once you have closed the lid of the machine.
4. Remove dough from bread machine when cycle is complete.
5. Set your oven to 350 degrees F and line a baking tray with parchment paper.
6. Flatten the dough and spread it on the prepared tray and bake for 5-7 minutes on each side or until browned.
7. Top with your favorite topping and return to the oven for about 3-5 more minutes or store it in the freezer for later use.

**Nutrition:** Calories 118, Total Fat 9 g, Carb 6, Dietary Fiber 3 g, Protein 5 g, Cholesterol 27 mg, Sodium 116 mg

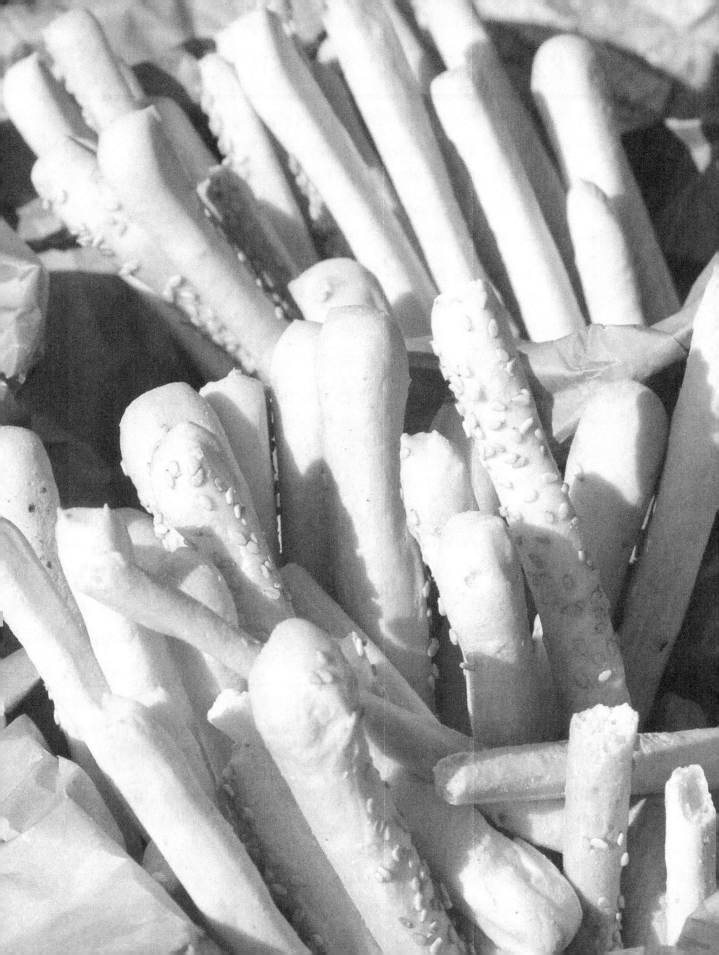

# 82. KETO BREADSTICKS BASE

## INGREDIENTS

- 2 cups Mozzarella Cheese (~8 oz.)
- ¾ cup Cheddar Cheese (~3 oz.)
- 3/4 cup Almond Flour
- 1 tbsp. Psyllium Husk Powder
- 3 tbsp. Cream Cheese (~1.5 oz.)
- 1 huge Egg
- 1 tsp. Preparing Powder

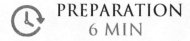 **PREPARATION** 6 MIN　　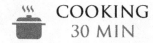 **COOKING** 30 MIN　　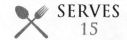 **SERVES** 15

## DIRECTIONS

1. Pre-heat stove to 400F.
2. Combine egg and cream cheddar until somewhat joined. In another bowl, consolidate all the dry fixings following order in your bread machine's manual instructions.
3. Measure out the mozzarella cheddar and microwave in 20-second interims until sizzling.
4. Add the egg, cream cheddar, and dry fixings into the mozzarella cheddar and combine.
5. Pour mixture in the bread machine loaf pan.
6. Place the bread pan in the machine, and select the breadstick setting. If not available use cookies or pasta dough program.
7. Then press start once you have closed the lid of the machine.
8. Remove dough from bread machine when cycle is complete.
9. Divide the dough into 15 equal pieces and roll them with your hands forming breadsticks.

10. At that point season the mixture with the flavorings you like.

11. Arrange the breadsticks on the baking sheet and brush them with the egg yolks.

12. Bake 13-15 minutes on top rack until fresh.

13. Serve while warm!

**Nutrition:** Cal 60, Carb 4 g, Net Carb 2.5 g, Fiber 4.5 g, Fat 6 g, Protein 4 g, Sugars 3 g

# 83. ALMOND FLOUR BREADSTICKS

## INGREDIENTS

**For Breadstick:**
- 2 eggs
- 1 ½ tbsp. Olive oil
- ½ tsp. Oregano
- ½ tsp. Parsley
- ½ tsp. Basil
- ½ tsp. Garlic powder
- ½ tsp. Onion powder
- 2 ½ tbsp. Coconut flour
- 2 cups almond flour

**For Topping:**
- ¼ tsp. Salt
- ½ tsp. Garlic powder
- 2 tsp. Parmesan grated
- 1 tbsp. Olive oil

 **PREPARATION** 5 MIN

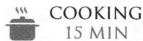 **COOKING** 15 MIN

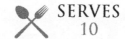 **SERVES** 10

## DIRECTIONS

1. Preheat the oven to 350 F and line a baking pan with parchment paper.
2. In a bowl, whisk almond flour, olive oil, and seasoning.
3. Whisk the eggs in another bowl, mix into the almond flour.
4. Add 1 tbsp. Coconut flour to the mixture at a time, stirring to combine.
5. Allow dough to rest for 1 to 2 minutes after each tbsp. Once the mixture gets thick, add the remaining coconut flour.
6. Pour mixture in the bread machine loaf pan.
7. Place the bread pan in the machine, and select the breadstick setting. If not available use cookies or pasta dough program.
8. Then press start once you have closed the lid of the machine.
9. Remove dough from bread machine when cycle is complete.
10. Form dough into a ball. And roll out into 1.5-inch wide rope-like sticks.

11. Transfer to the prepared baking sheet, place in the oven, and bake for 10 minutes.
12. Meanwhile, mix together salt, parmesan, and garlic.
13. Once baked, carefully brush the tops of breadsticks with oil, then sprinkle with garlic parmesan mix.
14. Bake for 5 minutes more.

**Nutrition:** Calories 169, Fat 15 g, Carb 6.14 g, Protein 7 g

# 84. CHEESY BREADSTICKS

## INGREDIENTS

**For breadsticks:**
- ½ cup of parmesan cheese, shredded
- 1 cups of mozzarella cheese, shredded
- ½ teaspoon of garlic powder
- 1 teaspoon of Italian seasoning
- ¼ teaspoon of baking powder
- ½ teaspoon of salt

- 4 eggs
- 1 oz of cream cheese, softened
- 1/3 cup of coconut flour
- 4 ½ tablespoons of butter (melted and cooled)

**For topping:**
- 12 teaspoons of Italian seasoning
- ¼ cup of parmesan cheese, shredded

 **PREPARATION** 10 MIN

 **COOKING** 15 MIN

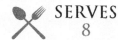 **SERVES** 8

## DIRECTIONS

1. Preheat your oven to 400 degrees F.
2. Prepare a 7x11 baking pan by greasing it with cooking spray.
3. Combine the cream cheese, salt, eggs and melted butter then mix.
4. Add the spices, baking powder and coconut flour to the butter mixture and stir until combined then stir in the parmesan and mozzarella.
5. Pour mixture in the bread machine loaf pan.
6. Place the bread pan in the machine, and select the breadstick setting. If not available use cookies or pasta dough program.
7. Then press start once you have closed the lid of the machine.
8. Remove dough from bread machine when cycle is complete.
9. Transfer the batter to a casserole dish then top with the additional Italian spices, parmesan cheese and mozzarella.
10. Bake until the breadsticks are done for 15 minutes. Halfway through baking, use a pizza cutter to create individual breadsticks.
11. Transfer the pan to the top rack of your oven and broil until the cheese is bubbly and brown for around 1-2 minutes
12. Serve with keto friendly marinara sauce.

**Nutrition:** Calories 299, Protein 17 g, Carb 4 g, Fat 23 g

# 85. ITALIAN BREADSTICKS

## INGREDIENTS

- 1 tbsp. of pulverized psyllium husk
- 3/4 cup of almond flour
- 1 tbsp. of flaxseed meal
- 3 tbsp. of cream cheese
- 1 tsp. baking powder—gluten-free
- 2 cups mozzarella cheese—shredded
- 2 medium eggs
- 1 tsp. of pepper
- 2 tsp. of Italian seasoning
- 1 tsp. of salt

 **PREPARATION**
10 MIN

 **COOKING**
20 MIN

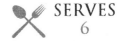 **SERVES**
6

## DIRECTIONS

1. Make sure that the oven is set to heat at 400°F. Use a silicone baking mat or cover a standard sized baking sheet with baking paper.
2. Place 2 pieces of parchment paper to the side or you can use aluminum foil instead.
3. On medium heat, use a double boiler to melt the mozzarella cheese completely.
4. Meanwhile, in another bowl, combine the eggs and cream cheese until mixed thoroughly. Set to the side.
5. Whisk the psyllium husk & baking powders & almond flour into the large-sized bowl together, removing any lumps.
6. Add in the mixture of cheese to the bowl of dry ingredient and mix thoroughly. Next, add the melted mozzarella cheese to the batter.
7. Pour mixture in the bread machine loaf pan.
8. Place the bread pan in the machine, and select the breadstick setting. If not available use cookies or pasta dough program.
9. Then press start once you have closed the lid of the machine.

10. Remove dough from bread machine when cycle is complete.
11. Use a rolling pin to press the dough flat on parchment paper, keeping an even thickness throughout.
12. Transfer the flattened dough to a piece of aluminum foil or the additional piece of parchment paper to cut into strips with a pizza cutter.
13. Sprinkle the salt, Italian seasoning and pepper on each breadstick.
14. Put it on a piece of cookie sheet & then you need to bake it for 13-15 mins. and serve warm.

**Nutrition:** Calories 238, Net Carb 2.8 g, Fat 19 g, Protein 13 g

# 86. ULTIMATE KETO BREADSTICKS

## INGREDIENTS

**For breadsticks:**
- ¼ cup coconut flour
- ¾ cup ground flax seeds
- 1 tbsp. psyllium husk powder
- 1 cup almond flour
- 2 tbsp. ground chia seeds
- 1 tsp. salt
- 1 cup lukewarm water, plus more if needed

**For topping:**
- 2 egg yolks, for brushing
- 4 tbsp. mixed seeds
- 1 tsp. coarse sea salt

 **PREPARATION** 10 MIN

 **COOKING** 40 MIN

 **SERVES** 20

## DIRECTIONS

1. Preheat the oven to 350F.
2. Combine the almond flour, psyllium husks, flax seeds, and coconut flour to bread machine pan following order in your bread machine's manual instructions. Add the chia seeds, salt, and the water.
3. Place the bread pan in the machine, and select the breadstick setting. If not available use cookies or pasta dough program.
4. Then press start once you have closed the lid of the machine.
5. Remove dough from bread machine when cycle is complete.
6. Cover and place in the fridge for 20-30 minutes.
7. Line a baking sheet with parchment paper.
8. Divide the dough into 20 equal pieces and roll them with your hands forming breadsticks.
9. Arrange the breadsticks on the baking sheet and brush them with the egg yolks.
10. Sprinkle with seeds and salt and bake for 20 minutes.
11. Serve.

**Nutrition:** Calories 75, Fat 9.6 g, Carb 4.1 g, Protein 3.5 g

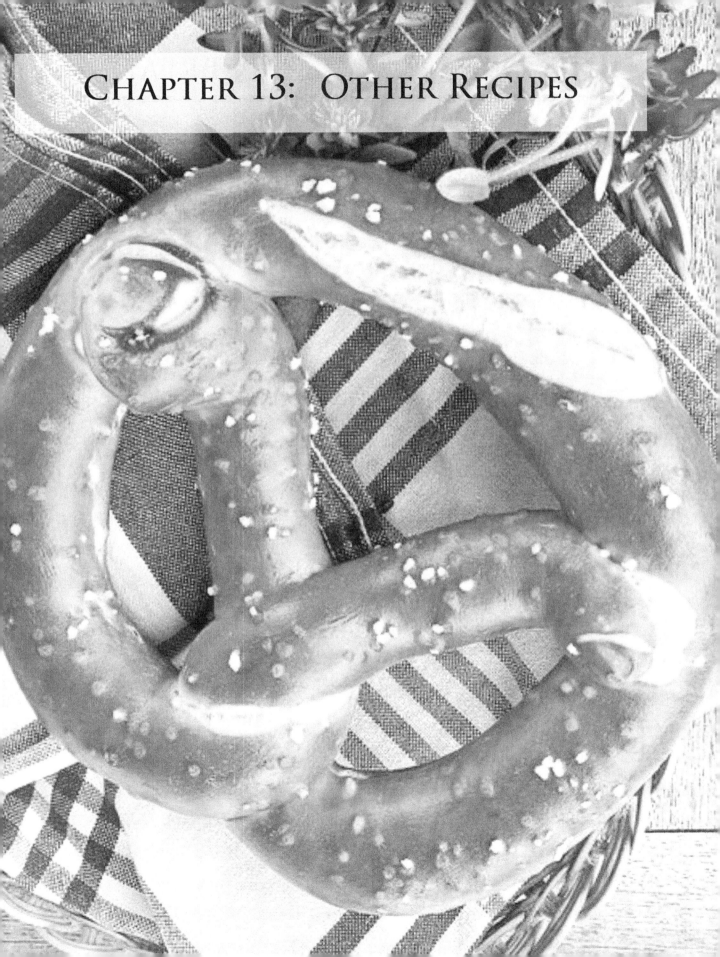

# CHAPTER 13: OTHER RECIPES

# 87. PUMPKIN PECAN BREAD

## INGREDIENTS

- ½ cup almond milk
- ½ cup canned pumpkin
- 1 egg
- 2 tablespoons margarine or butter, cut up
- 3 cups almond flour
- 3 tablespoons erythritol
- 1 tablespoon inulin
- ¾ tsp salt
- ¼ tsp ground nutmeg
- ¼ tsp ground ginger
- 1/8 tsp ground cloves
- 1 tsp active dry yeast or bread machine yeast
- ¾ cup coarsely chopped pecans

 **PREPARATION** 10 MIN

 **COOKING** 3 HOURS

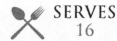 **SERVES** 16

## DIRECTIONS

1. Add ingredients to bread machine pan following bread machine's manual instructions, taking care on how to mix in the yeast.
2. Place the bread pan in the machine, and select the basic bread setting, together with the bread size and light/medium crust type, if available, then press start once you have closed the lid of the machine.
3. When the bread is ready, using oven mitts, remove the bread pan from the machine.
4. Use a stainless spatula to extract the bread from the pan and turn the pan upside down on a metallic rack where the bread will cool off before slicing it.

**Nutrition:** Calories 183, Fat 12 g sat. fat), Sodium 126 mg, Carb 7 g, Fiber 2 g, Protein 6.5 g

# 88. RED HOT CINNAMON BREAD

## INGREDIENTS

- ¼ cup lukewarm water
- ½ cup lukewarm almond milk
- ¼ cup softened butter
- 2 ¼ tsp instant yeast
- 1 ¼ tsp salt
- ¼ cup Swerve
- 1 teaspoon honey or sugar (or Inulin)
- 1 tsp vanilla
- 1 large egg, lightly beaten
- 3 cups almond flour
- ½ cup Cinnamon Red Hot candies

 **PREPARATION** 5 MIN      **COOKING** 3 MIN     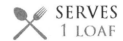 **SERVES** 1 LOAF

## DIRECTIONS

1. Add ingredients to bread machine pan except candy.
2. Choose dough setting.
3. After cycle is over, turn dough out into bowl and cover, let rise for 45 minutes to one hour.
4. Gently punch down dough and shape into a rectangle.
5. Knead in the cinnamon candies in 1/3 at a t time.
6. Shape the dough into a loaf and place in a greased or parchment lined loaf pan.
7. Tent the pan loosely with lightly greased plastic wrap, and allow a second rise for 40-50 minutes.
8. Preheat oven 350 degrees.
9. Bake 30-40 minutes.
10. Remove and cool on wire rack before slicing.

**Nutrition:** Calories 207, Total fat 6.9 g (4.1 g sat. fat), Sodium 317 mg, Carb 4 g, Fiber 1 g, Protein 7.6 g

# 89. HEARTY SEEDED BREAD LOAF

## INGREDIENTS

- ½ cups pumpkin seeds (1 cup finely chopped with a food processor)
- ½ cup whole psyllium husks
- ½ cup flax seeds
- ½ cup chia seeds
- ½ cups warm water
- 1 tsp. pink salt
- 1 cup raw sunflower seeds
- 1 tbsp. sugar-free maple syrup
- 1 tbsp. melted coconut oil

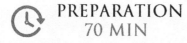 **PREPARATION** 70 MIN    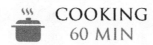 **COOKING** 60 MIN    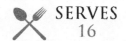 **SERVES** 16

## DIRECTIONS

1. Prepare bread machine loaf pan greasing it with cooking spray.
2. In a bowl, mix together dry Ingredients until well combined.
3. Pour the maple syrup, warm water, and melted coconut oil into another bowl and continue stirring until the batter becomes thick.
4. Following the instructions on your machine's manual, mix the dry ingredients into the wet ingredients and pour in the bread machine loaf pan, taking care to follow how to mix in the baking powder.
5. Place the bread pan in the machine, and select the basic bread setting, together with the bread size, if available, then press start once you have closed the lid of the machine.
6. When the bread is ready, using oven mitts, remove the bread pan from the machine.
7. Let it cool before slicing.
8. Cool, slice, and serve.

**Nutrition:** Calories 172, Fat 6 g, Carb 2 g, Protein 7 g

# 90. EGGY COCONUT BREAD

## INGREDIENTS

- ½ cup coconut flour
- 4 eggs
- 1 cup water
- 1 tbsp. apple cider vinegar
- ¼ cup coconut oil, plus 1 tsp. melted
- ½ tsp. garlic powder
- ½ tsp. baking soda
- ¼ tsp. salt

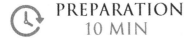 **PREPARATION** 10 MIN     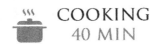 **COOKING** 40 MIN     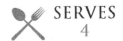 **SERVES** 4

## DIRECTIONS

1. Prepare bread machine loaf pan greasing it with cooking spray.
2. In a bowl, mix together coconut flour, baking soda, garlic powder, and salt. Until well combined.
3. Into another bowl, add eggs to a blender along with vinegar, water, and ¼-cup coconut oil. Blend for 30 seconds.
4. Following the instructions on your machine's manual, mix the dry ingredients into the wet ingredients and pour in the bread machine loaf pan, taking care to follow how to mix in the baking powder.
5. Place the bread pan in the machine, and select the basic bread setting, together with the bread size and crust type, if available, then press start once you have closed the lid of the machine.
6. When the bread is ready, using oven mitts, remove the bread pan from the machine.
7. Let it cool before slicing.
8. Cool, slice, and enjoy.

**Nutrition:** Calories 297, Fat 14 g, Carb 9 g, Protein 15 g

# 91. SPICY BREAD

## INGREDIENTS

- ½ cup coconut flour
- 6 eggs
- 3 large jalapenos, sliced
- 4 ounces turkey bacon, sliced
- ½ cup ghee
- ¼ tsp. baking soda
- ¼ tsp. salt
- ¼ cup water

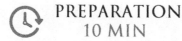 **PREPARATION** 10 MIN

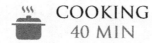 **COOKING** 40 MIN

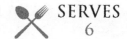 **SERVES** 6

## DIRECTIONS

1. Cut bacon and jalapenos on a baking tray and roast for 10 minutes.
2. Flip and bake for 5 more minutes.
3. Remove seeds from the jalapenos.
4. Place jalapenos and bacon slices in a food processor and blend until smooth.
5. In a bowl, mix together add the coconut flour, baking soda, and salt. Stir until well combined.
6. Into another bowl, add ghee, eggs, and ¼-cup water. Mix well.
7. Add bacon and jalapeno mix.
8. Grease the machine loaf pan with ghee.
9. Following the instructions on your machine's manual, mix the dry ingredients into the wet ingredients and pour in the bread machine loaf pan, taking care to follow how to mix in the baking powder.
10. Place the bread pan in the machine, and select the basic bread setting, together with the bread size and crust type, if available, then press start once you have closed the lid of the machine.
11. When the bread is ready, using oven mitts, remove the bread pan from the machine.
12. Let it cool before slicing.

**Nutrition:** Calories 240, Fat 20 g, Carb 5 g, Protein 9 g

# 92. CHOCOLATE CHIP SCONES

## INGREDIENTS

- 2 cups almond flour
- 1 tsp. baking soda
- ¼ tsp. sea salt
- 1 egg
- 2 tbsp. low-carb sweetener
- 2 tbsp. milk, cream or yogurt
- ½ cup sugar-free chocolate chips

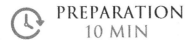 **PREPARATION**
10 MIN

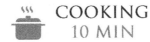 **COOKING**
10 MIN

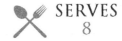 **SERVES**
8

## DIRECTIONS

1. Preheat the oven to 350F.
2. In a bowl, add almond flour, baking soda, and salt and blend.
3. Then add the egg, sweetener, milk, and chocolate chips. Blend well.
4. Pour mixture in the bread machine loaf pan.
5. Place the bread pan in the machine, and select the cookies setting. If not available use pasta dough program.
6. Then press start once you have closed the lid of the machine.
7. Remove dough from bread machine when cycle is complete.
8. Pat the dough into a ball and place it on parchment paper.
9. Roll the dough with a rolling pin into a large circle. Slice it into 8 triangular pieces.
10. Place the scones and parchment paper on a baking sheet and separate the scones about 1 inch or so apart.
11. Bake for 7 to 10 minutes or until lightly browned.
12. Cool and serve.

**Nutrition:** Calories 213, Fat 18 g, Carb 10 g, Protein 8 g

# 93. FATHEAD ROLLS

## INGREDIENTS

- ¾ cup shredded mozzarella cheese
- 3 oz. cream cheese
- ½ cup shredded cheddar cheese
- 2 beaten egg
- ¼ tsp. garlic powder
- 1/3 cup almond flour
- 2 tsp. baking powder

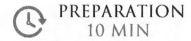 **PREPARATION** 10 MIN

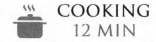 **COOKING** 12 MIN

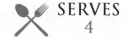 **SERVES** 4

## DIRECTIONS

1. Preheat the oven to 425F.
2. Combine the cream cheese and mozzarella. Place in the microwave and cook for 20 seconds at a time until cheese melts.
3. Beat the eggs in another bowl, add all the dry ingredients (set aside 1.5 tablespoons of almond flour) and stir in cheddar cheese.
4. Pour the mixture into bread machine pan following order in your bread machine's manual instructions.
5. Place the bread pan in the machine, and select the dough program.
6. Then press start once you have closed the lid of the machine.
7. Remove dough from bread machine when cycle is complete.
8. Gently start working the dough into a ball. Cover and place in the fridge for ½ hour.
9. Sprinkle the top of the bread with remaining almond flour.

10. Slice the dough ball into four parts and roll each one into a ball. Cut the ball in half.

11. Place the cut side down onto a well-greased sheet pan.
12. Bake for 10 to 12 minutes.

**Nutrition:** Calories 160, Fat 13 g, Carb 2.5 g, Protein 7 g

# 94. LOW-CARB PRETZELS

## INGREDIENTS

- 1 tbsp. pretzel salt
- 2 tbsp. butter, melted
- 2 tbsp. warm water
- 2 tsp. dried yeast
- 2 eggs
- 2 tsp. xanthan gum
- 1 ½ cups almond flour
- 4 tbsp. cream cheese
- 3 cups of shredded mozzarella cheese

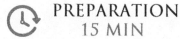 **PREPARATION** 15 MIN

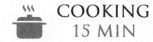 **COOKING** 15 MIN

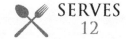 **SERVES** 12

## DIRECTIONS

1. Preheat the oven to 390F.
2. Melt the mozzarella cheese and cream cheese in the microwave.
3. Mix the almond meal and xanthan gum with a hand mixer.
4. Add all ingredients to bread machine pan following order in your bread machine's manual instructions, taking care on how to mix in the yeast.
5. Place the bread pan in the machine, and select the dough cycle setting.
6. Then press start once you have closed the lid of the machine.
7. Remove dough from bread machine when cycle is complete.
8. Divide into 12 balls while the dough is still warm, then roll into a long, thin log and then twist to form a pretzel shape.
9. Cover a large cookie sheet with parchment paper.
10. Transfer onto a lined cookie sheet, leaving small space between them.
11. Brush the remaining butter on top the pretzels and sprinkle with the salt.
12. Bake for 12 to 15 minutes in the oven or until golden brown.

**Nutrition:** Calories 217, Fat 18 g, Carb: 3 g, Protein 11 g

# 95. IRANIAN FLAT BREAD (SANGAK)

## INGREDIENTS

- 4 cups almond flour
- 2 ½ cups warm water
- 1 tbsp. instant yeast
- 12 tsp. sesame seeds
- Salt to taste

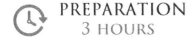 **PREPARATION** 3 HOURS

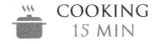 **COOKING** 15 MIN

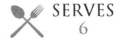 **SERVES** 6

## DIRECTIONS

1. Add all ingredients to bread machine pan following order in your bread machine's manual instructions, taking care on how to mix in the yeast.
2. Place the bread pan in the machine, and select the dough cycle setting.
3. Then press start once you have closed the lid of the machine.
4. Remove dough from bread machine when cycle is complete.
5. Shape the dough into a ball and let stand for 3 hours covered.
6. Preheat the oven to 480F.
7. With a rolling pin, roll out the dough, and divide into 6 balls.
8. Roll each ball into ½ inch thick rounds.
9. Line a baking sheet with parchment paper and place the rolled rounds on it.
10. With a finger, make a small hole in the middle and add 2 tsp sesame seeds in each hole.
11. Bake for 3 to 4 minutes, then flip over and bake for 2 minutes more.
12. Serve.

**Nutrition:** Calories 26, Fat 1 g, Carb 3.5 g, Protein 0.7 g

# 96. SNICKERDOODLES

## INGREDIENTS

- 2 cups almond flour
- 2 tbsp. coconut flour
- ¼ tsp. baking soda
- ¼ tsp. salt
- 3 tbsp. unsalted butter, melted
- 1/3 cup low-carb sweetener
- ¼ cup coconut milk
- 1 tbsp. vanilla extract
- 2 tbsp. ground cinnamon
- 2 tbsp. low-carb granulated sweetener

 **PREPARATION** 10 MIN     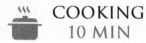 **COOKING** 10 MIN     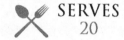 **SERVES** 20

## DIRECTIONS

1. Preheat the oven to 350F.
2. Whisk together the coconut flour, almond flour, baking soda, and salt in a bowl.
3. In another bowl, cream the butter, sweetener, milk and vanilla.
4. Add all ingredients to bread machine pan following order in your bread machine's manual instructions.
5. Place the bread pan in the machine, and select the cookies dough setting. If not available use pasta dough program.
6. Then press start once you have closed the lid of the machine.
7. Remove dough from bread machine when cycle is complete.
8. Line baking sheets with parchment paper.
9. Blend the ground cinnamon and low-carb granulated sweetener together in a bowl. With your hands, roll a tbsp. of dough into a ball.
10. Roll the dough ball in the cinnamon mixture to fully coat.

11. Place the dough balls on the cookie sheet, spread about an inch apart, and flatten with the underside of a jar.

12. Bake for 8 to 10 minutes.

13. Cool and serve.

**Nutrition:** Calories 86, Fat 7 g, Carb 3 g, Protein 3 g

# 97. PARMESAN-THYME POPOVERS

## INGREDIENTS

- 4 eggs
- ½ cup coconut milk
- 2 tbsp. coconut flour
- Pinch salt
- 1 tbsp. parmesan cheese
- 1 tbsp. chopped fresh thyme

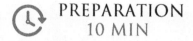 **PREPARATION** 10 MIN

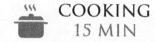 **COOKING** 15 MIN

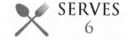 **SERVES** 6

## DIRECTIONS

1. Preheat the oven to 425F.
2. Pre-grease a 12 cupcake pan with butter or oil
3. Add all ingredients to bread machine pan following order in your bread machine's manual instructions.
4. Place the bread pan in the machine, and select the cookies dough setting. If not available use pasta dough program.
5. Then press start once you have closed the lid of the machine.
6. Remove dough from bread machine when cycle is complete.
7. Fill greased nonstick cupcake pan at 2/3 level with dough.
8. Bake for 15 minutes, or until they begin to brown on top.
9. Cool and serve.

**Nutrition:** Calories 64, Fat 34 g, Carb 2 g, Protein 3 g

# 98. KETO-BREAD TWISTS

## INGREDIENTS

- ¼ cup almond flour
- 2 tbsp. coconut flour
- ½ tsp. salt
- ½ tbsp. baking powder
- ½ cup cheese, shredded
- 2 tbsp. butter
- 2 eggs
- ¼ cup green pesto

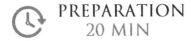 **PREPARATION** 20 MIN

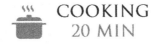 **COOKING** 20 MIN

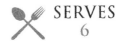 **SERVES** 6

## DIRECTIONS

1. Preheat the oven to 350F and prepare a baking tray.
2. Combine coconut flour, almond flour, baking powder, and salt in a bowl.
3. Mix butter, cheese, and egg in another bowl.
4. Combine the flour mixture with the butter mixture pour it to bread machine pan following order in your bread machine's manual instructions.
5. Place the bread pan in the machine, and select the cookies dough setting. If not available use pasta dough program.
6. Then press start once you have closed the lid of the machine.
7. Remove dough from bread machine when cycle is complete.
8. Take 2 parchment sheets and place the dough in between them.
9. Form the dough into a rectangular shape with a rolling pin and remove the parchment paper from one side.
10. Drizzle the green pesto on the loaf and cut it into strips and twist them.
11. Put the baking tray in the oven and bake for 20 minutes.
12. Remove from oven and serve.

**Nutrition:** Calories 151, Fat 12.9 g, Carb 3.5 g, Protein 5.8 g

# 99. MUSTARD BEER BREAD

## INGREDIENTS

- 1 ¼ cups dark beer
- 2 1/3 cups almond flour
- ¾ cup whole almond meal
- 1 tablespoon olive oil
- 3 teaspoons mustard seeds
- 1 ½ teaspoons dry yeast
- 1 teaspoon salt
- 2 teaspoons brown sugar

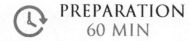 **PREPARATION** 60 MIN   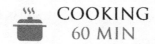 **COOKING** 60 MIN   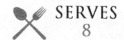 **SERVES** 8

## DIRECTIONS

1. Open a bottle of beer and let it stand for 30 minutes to get out the gas.
2. In a bread maker's bucket, add the beer, mustard seeds, butter, amond flour, and almond meal.
3. From different angles in the bucket, put salt and sugar. In the center of the flour, make a groove and fill with the mustard seeds.
4. Start the baking program.
5. When cycle in finished and bread in ready, remove it from the pan and let cool in a banneton.
6. Enjoy!

**Nutrition:** Calories 148, Carbohydrates 4.2 g, Fats 21 g, Protein 4.1 g

# 100.   LIKE-POTATO ROSEMARY KETO-BREAD

## INGREDIENTS

- 3 jicama root  (like potatoes replacement)
- 4 cups almond flour
- 1 tablespoon sugar (needed to activate yeast)
- 1 tablespoon oil
- 3 ½ teaspoons salt
- 1 ½ cups water
- 1 teaspoon dry yeast
- 1 cup mashed potatoes, ground through a sieve
- crushed rosemary

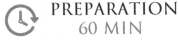 **PREPARATION** 60 MIN    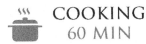 **COOKING** 60 MIN    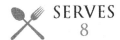 **SERVES** 8

## DIRECTIONS

1. Peel the jicama root and shred it using a food processor.
2. Place the shredded jicama root in a colander to allow the water to drain. Mix in 2 tsp of salt as well.
3. Squeeze out the remaining liquid.
4. Microwave the shredded jicama for 5-8 minutes. This step pre-cooks it.
5. Measure the required amount of ingredients. Install the mixing paddle in the baking container.
6. Fill with flour, remaining salt, and sugar.
7. Add sunflower oil and water.
8. Close the lid, and put the yeast in the specially designated hole.
9. Set the mode of baking bread with a filling, according to the instructions of the bread maker.
10. When the dough knits and comes up the right number of times, a beep will sound, which means that you can add additional ingredients. Open the lid of the bread maker and pour in the jicama mixture and chopped rosemary. Close and press the "Start" button.
11. After the oven is finished, immediately remove the bread from the baking container.
12. Let cool down.
13. Serve and enjoy.

**Nutrition:** Calories 276, Carbohydrates 5 g, Fats 2.8 g, Protein 7.4 g

# 101. HOMEMADE OMEGA-3 BREAD

## INGREDIENTS

- 3/5 cup almond milk
- ½ cup water
- 2 eggs
- 2 tablespoons rapeseed oil
- 3 cups almond flour
- 1 cup flax flour
- 2 teaspoons dry yeast
- 2 teaspoons salt
- 1 tablespoons cane sugar (needed for yeast activation)

- 3 tablespoons flaxseeds
- 1 tablespoon sesame seeds

---

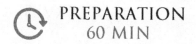 **PREPARATION**
60 MIN

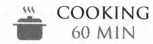 **COOKING**
60 MIN

**SERVES**
8

## DIRECTIONS

1. Soak the flaxseeds in cool water for 30 minutes.
2. Combine all the liquid ingredients in the bread pan
3. Add sifted almond flour, flaxseed flour, yeast, sugar, and salt.
4. Set it to the Basic program.
5. After the signal sounds, remove from pan
6. Add sesame seeds and strained flaxseeds.

**Nutrition:** Calories 289, Carbohydrates 4.5 g, Fats 9 g, Protein 11.1 g

# CONCLUSION

Thank you for reaching the end of this book. A bread machine and this book is really a perfect couple in your kitchen. Finally, you can have lots of choices of keto bread you can make and serve for your beloved ones.

Bread is staple food that is consumed daily. Since health is the first number of investments in life, it is a good thing if you can prepare it from home. That means everything contained in the bread you and your beloved eat almost every day is under control.

Every recipe in this book is specially created for those who concern not only to health but also taste. However, consume the keto bread with several additional nourishing food, such as vegetables, meat, cheese, and many other healthy food options is totally great since it will enhance the nutritious content of the food.

For sure, every single recipe in this book has been tried in our kitchen and all of them are superb. However, as practice always makes perfect, it is suggested to you to make the bread as often as possible and to engage with your bread machine.

Cutting a lot of foods that are favorites is one of the main struggles that people go through when on keto diet.

Concentrate on the positives and you will succeed. Keto diet helps in prevention of some diseases such as respiratory problems, heart diseases and diabetes.

It does not matter if you want to start the keto lifestyle yourself or you are in search of traditional bread, there are suitable recipes for your every need. They range from sweet to savory and they are healthy and so satisfying. There is little effort needed to make these recipes using the bread machine.

Have wonderful and amazing experiences with your bread machine and enjoy baking, healthy people!

Made in the USA
Coppell, TX
23 February 2025

46301998R10116